Exploring Education

Sex Education
in School and Society

Dorothy M. Dallas
Lecturer in Education, King's College, London

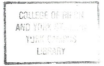
NFER

Published by the National Foundation for Education Research
in England and Wales

Registered Office: The Mere, Upton Park, Slough, Bucks, SL1 2DQ

Book Publishing Division: 2 Jennings Buildings, Thames Avenue,
Windsor, Berks, SL4 1QS

First Published 1972

SBN 901225 91 6

Cover design by
PETER GAULD, FSIA

Printed in Great Britain by
KING, THORNE & STACE LTD., SCHOOL ROAD, HOVE, BN3 5JE

Contents

Acknowledgements

To Derek Lewis, Adviser in Health Education to the City of Oxford Education Committee, for his many detailed comments and useful additions after reading the first draft of this book.

To Jill Davies, Organizing Lecturer, London Diocesan Committee for Personal Relationships, for reading and commenting on the first draft.

To the Nuffield Foundation, for facilities given in connection with the Secondary Science Project, to discuss the problems and methods of sex education with over 2,000 teachers in England, Wales and Northern Ireland; also to Mrs. Misselbrook, the Project Organizer, and W. Anderson, Publications Editor, for much helpful criticism and advice.

To Gabriel Chanan, the Editor, for help with the manuscript.

To Dr. C. S. Nicol, Lydia Department, St. Thomas Hospital, London, for, among other things, advice on the section dealing with VD.

To F. St. D. Rowntree, Health Education Officer, City of Sheffield; Pat Parrish, Health Education Officer, Carshalton, and to Richard and Hepzibah Hauser for permission to publish private communications.

To Michael Schofield and the Health Education Council Ltd., Peter McPhail, the Schools Council and Longmans for permission to extract from unpublished works.

To John Wilson, David Barnard, Dr. Tunnadine and the Family Planning Association, for permission to publish extracts of their books.

To the BBC Schools Broadcasting Council and Grampian TV, for permission to publish findings from their evaluations of programmes.

To Veronica Armstrong for the graphics on pages 88–9.

Finally, to Mrs. Val Saunders for typing the manuscript.

A recent review of sex education said that it was almost non-existent in Britain; it does exist but on the whole prefers to shun publicity and sensational comment from superficial appraisers.

For this reason, names of individual schools are omitted from this text, but genuine professional inquiries will be passed on to the school concerned by the author.

CHAPTER ONE

Objectives

Objectives in sex education
SEX EDUCATION is a wide, all embracing and all but meaningless term; various synonyms have been coined and employed, but have failed to replace it in common usage. Its interpretation has become sharply polarized; on the one hand it is associated with anatomical diagrams and bald explanations of physiological processes, while on the other the vaguer realms of 'personal relationships' are explored. It is not common to find the two approaches integrated; usually they exist side by side and in watertight compartments, largely because those who feel securely expert in one approach feel very inadequate in the other. This is one of the factors behind the rising number of adolescent school children who complain that they have too much sex education—a South London girl said that she had 'done' VD in biology, in religious instruction and in English lessons—and now the Local Authority Health Educators were coming in to 'do' it again! While one can understand the desire of the girl's individual teachers to ensure that she has certain essential knowledge it would seem likely that an interdisciplinary and co-ordinated approach might have answered some of her questions rather more to her satisfaction. Also it seems a pity that so much time had been spent on one aspect of sex education when many others had been left out completely.

Hence the need for the close examination of objectives in sex education; since we are irrevocably stuck with the term, it needs clarification and an extension of its meaning, especially as an interdisciplinary exercise.

Yesterday's objectives in sex education
The belief prevalent in the early part of the twentieth century, that sex education of the intelligent adolescent was best served by one short, sharp talk—in the fifth if the school was enlightened, in the sixth if it was felt to be an unpleasant but unavoidable duty—

was perhaps typical of attitudes to education in many other disciplines. Facts were enough, and sex was put over in a way similar to that used when dealing with the maps of the coalfields. The only difference was the special atmosphere which surrounded the short, sharp talk. It must often have conveyed to its victims that these matters were unspeakable and that no well-bred pupil would either need or dare to investigate them further. This method had at least one advantage—it did not attract unfavourable criticism from parents or education committees, largely because all concerned were much too embarrassed to mention it.

After the First World War, pragmatic objectives in sex education became more apparent, and, by the early 1930's, several of our national agencies concerned with the prevention of illegitimacy, the spread of knowledge about contraceptives and marriage guidance had begun. There was a small but interesting upsurge of intellectuals, who nobly hid their embarrassment as they discussed sexual matters with their children and solemnly left the bathroom door unlocked so that nudity could be rationally displayed.

There were, however, even in those days, teachers in schools effectively relieving adolescent anxiety and ignorance about sex often under the name of human biology, with equivocally worded syllabuses, and without a word to the head. Such strategies are still in use today. Cyril Bibby, the doyen of sex educators in this country, was by the late 1930's experienced enough to write his excellent books. These were sufficiently unsensational to be put into many public libraries and so improved the traditional method of sex education of the middle class adolescent. (Until the recent increase in the public debate on sex education, the middle class child sex-educated himself from books, and had relatively little access to someone with whom he could discuss what he had read.)

Nevertheless, from the thirties up to the present day, too many schools practised the type of sex education lesson so clearly outlined in John Wilson's *Logic and Sexual Morality* (1965). Wilson's description shows a typical biologist's approach, together with the unvoiced comments of the class, and provides a warning that feedback and evaluation are as essential in sex education as in algebra.

The historical roots of embarrassment felt when talking about sex are a fascinating problem and a PhD awaits someone who

10

investigates them thoroughly. What happened to the bawdy but honest climate of dialogue of Restoration times? What changed it into the dual morality of Victorian times? What part did the apes and angels debate, Darwin, Huxley, take in shaping public attitudes towards the rejection of animality?

Negative objectives

With the Second World War in 1939 came the realization that there was a need for sex education for the Armed Forces, particularly about venereal diseases (VD). For centuries armies had accepted that their fighting strength would be reduced considerably by the ravages of the spirochaete (Treponema pallidum) and the wily gonococcus. In Lewis and Clarke's journals of their expedition across the Rocky Mountains in the nineteenth century, it was taken for granted that the men would suffer from venereal diseases, just as the British take it for granted today that they will suffer from toothache, headache, or mosquito bites.

The changing nature of war, the enormous numbers involved, and more humane attitudes about war disability pensions, coupled perhaps with pay deductions for soldiers with VD, made education on this subject essential. Unfortunately the instruction provided in response to this need was not education, it was a form of training relying for the most part of instilling fear into the troops. Few members of the forces will forget those VD films—they had great visual impact, and for decades after these images have been retained with remarkable clarity.

'The ironic evidence from research on the effects of fear-arousing information in connection with . . . types of preventive health behaviour is that people tend to reject the information rather than change their behaviour (Radelfinger, 1965; Young, 1967). Fear sets up a need for coping with fear. It is generally easier to cope by disregarding or avoiding the information or rejecting the knowledge than by changing one's behaviour patterns' (Green, 1970).

While it is unrealistic to expect generals in the middle of total war to sit down and think seriously about VD education, we have no such excuse today. There are still advocates of the horror film approach, plus the admonitory 'Don't' in the field of drug addiction, although less so now in sex education; such negative methods only cope with the symptoms of the undesired behaviour without treating the underlying causes, or producing anything but a superficial change in attitudes. It is interesting but futile to speculate that if in 1940-5 the Armed Forces had really been educated about VD, perhaps the present enormous rise in VD cases among teenagers might have been prevented through education passed on by parents themselves.

But in the climate of discussion which existed when most of today's adolescents would have benefited from such knowledge, could anyone expect the ordinary British father to admit to his children that he had by his behaviour been at risk from VD? Or the ordinary British mother to admit to her daughters that she had been at risk with respect to an unwanted pregnancy, much less that she had had an abortion or even that she knew anything about contraceptives? Feelings of guilt and shame in the parent therefore combined with ignorance to make a conspiracy of silence.

When antibiotics were discovered and found to cure VD, the lack of education on their nature and mode of action resulted in todays' situation, where the growing resistance of organisms such as the gonococcus to antibiotics is commonplace. In the early days, soldiers realized with relief that VD could be cured, and a black market in antibiotics grew up in response to demand. Many VD victims took antibiotics without medical supervision and only until the symptoms disappeared, unaware that the bacteria which had survived were still living and breeding inside them. Years of such abuse have now made larger and larger doses of antibiotics essential for cure and it is a hard struggle for the research scientist to keep up with the discovery of new antibiotics to counter the effects of more and more resistant strains of bacteria.

Authoritarian training as opposed to education presupposes that the situation will not change (as it did with respect to VD) and that the general level of education of the recipients is low enough to admit total unquestioning acceptance of dogma. With today's high level of general education people will question any authority which seeks to prevent them from enjoying themselves or which tries to prevent their favourite form of relaxation/escapist behaviour. In addition the instigators of fear-inducing education show a lack of appreciation of basic human optimism and the disregard for

12

statistical probability which arises from it. Few people still smoking today believe that they will be one of the unlucky three out of five who will get cancer of the lung. Why should they not be in the category of the two who won't?

Similarly in sex education, all the knowledge in the world about contraceptives will not prevent some people from thinking that they will be the lucky ones, that those who do get pregnant are not only unlucky but probably foolish as well. So education must deal with the irrational aspects as well as the factual and conceptual matters.

So far, it would appear that it is the methods which are negative rather than the objectives; there would seem to be nothing negative in the desire to prevent VD, to stop illegitimate pregnancies, or to reduce family size[1] and so prevent over-population, until one compares these with some more positive objectives; for example, to educate people so that they may have stable and happy marriages, so that their relations with the opposite sex are based on knowledge, not on chance and insecure value judgements. The fact that the usage of the word intercourse has become so debased as to imply that physical sexual communication is all that is possible between the sexes indicates how far sex education in its most positive sense has yet to go, in the furtherance of what McPhail (Schools Council Moral Education Project) calls 'the considerate way of life' with its concommitant release of the individual from guilt and shame in these matters.

Today's objectives

Before we can establish a firm basis for deciding objectives in sex education, we need to clarify what is meant by morality (as opposed to moralizing), not least because the frequent criticism of such education is that it is, *per se*, immoral.

In Britain we are lucky to have had the work of John Wilson and the Farmington Trust for Research into Moral Education as a clear basis for thinking about morals. Wilson's work has been accepted with relief and delight by many workers in the field of sex education, and at least two curriculum reform projects have used his criteria

[1] Although in Sweden sex education was originally introduced to *increase* the birth rate. SJÖVALL (1969). In: *Responsible Parenthood and Sex Education.* IPPF.

for moral education as their basis: the Nuffield Secondary Science Project, with respect to the human life cycle and man's effect on his environment; and the Schools Council Moral Education Project, directed by Peter McPhail. A simple outline of Wilson's ideas is set out below. Those wishing more detailed information should consult Wilson (1970).

Wilson's criteria for the morally educated

1. Those who are morally educated have *equal concern* for the needs, feelings and interests of other people as they do for themselves.

2. To be able to have concern in such a way they must be *sensitive and perceptive to the needs of others*, perhaps even when the others are not aware of their own needs.

3. To be sensitive and perceptive they need *insight into human behaviour* and knowledge of factors involved in the production of one kind of behaviour rather than another.

4. Equal concern, sensitivity and knowledge of human behaviour are of little use if the morally educated person has not the *skills of both social and verbal communication* needed for action.

5. If all the above criteria are fulfilled, a morally educated person should be able to make *decisions about right and wrong*, within changing contexts, both for himself as an individual and for the various communities of which he holds membership.

6. Having made such decisions, the morally educated person is able to put into *action* the behaviour which he considers to be right.

7. It is impossible to achieve these criteria in certain fields where one is not *psychologically free*. An awareness of one's psychological handicaps is essential if loaded value judgements are not to be made.

Wilson's hypothesis provides a valuable analytical framework which has been used in several fields of health education as well as sex education; even if the aims formulated can never be absolutely achieved, it is obvious that they are well worth working towards. They can be used to aid much-needed assessments of the attitudes of teachers and parents and as guidelines in the moral education of the pupils in their general education as well as in sex education. It is worth while examining them in detail with respect to sex education as they provide comprehensive coverage of all its most debatable points.

Equal concern

To take equal and full concern for the needs of all others is a somewhat idealistic aim; the aim here in education is to widen the spectrum from self to all those involved when an individual makes a decision. Christ expressed it as 'Do unto others as you would have them do unto you', while Alex Comfort applied it specifically to sexual relations when he adjured us not to use another for selfish gratification of sexual needs. The Schools Council's Moral Education Project is concerned with promoting 'The considerate way of life', and so is the Nuffield Secondary Science Project, which applies this concept not only to sexual relations, but to the need for adolescents to understand other difficulties involved in growing to maturity. These include the search for identity, or, as Adler put it, for the secure self-image, and also the obligation to take equal concern for the needs of the elderly, for the unborn child and for the growing child.

It is the search for the secure self image which makes teaching about equal concern difficult with adolescents. An individual who feels inferior tends to look for someone else who can be regarded or treated as inferior to himself, to bolster up his sagging self-image. When the changing role of women, with their liberation from biological pressure of obligatory child bearing ('Liberation to do two jobs', as one disgruntled career girl put it), becomes a threat to male security of self-image, frustrated machismo can erupt as violence of all kinds. To take equal concern for all, and not only those who *appear* to be equals or superiors, is difficult in today's society in Britain.

Equal concern is the most central of Wilson's criteria. Many figures in world history have shown great sensitivity and perception of others' needs, have had a deep insight into the basis of human behaviour and have been able to make and to act upon judgements about right and wrong, but too often to the disadvantage of categories of people for whom they did not take an equal concern.

15

Sensitivity to the needs of others

How can one take concern for others if one has no idea of their needs? The one-shot sex education talk (see page 10) is a prime example of this; well-meaning people, often genuinely anxious to help the adolescent, may have little concept of their needs. A teacher in a Sussex school (in good communication with his class and aware of most of their needs), using the individual learning programme, *How Life Begins* (Reid and Booth, 1970), was nevertheless surprised by the flood of new questions from a class of 11-year-olds, when he repeated a section of the programme for the benefit of TV cameras; time to digest and assimilate had provided new synthesis of learning and new queries.

What are the needs of the various age, ability and cultural groups of children in sex education? Freedom from anxiety, guilt and shame has been paramount from very early days, although most people were originally concerned with sheer ignorance. An LCC publication *Some Notes on Sex Education* (1964) recommends 'A few words of reassurance on masturbation . . . given to boys of 13–14 to set this matter in proper perspective. The intention is that masturbation should not be seen as "a major sin or serious danger to health".' Anxieties created in young children by outside agencies, whether it is the dirty stories of schoolmates or the ideas about sex gained from advertising, appear to be international. A young Japanese girl is quoted as saying 'I felt unpleasant about sex when I saw obscene movie posters. Now I am quite refreshed by these slides since this shows sex exactly as I hope it would be—splendid.' (The slides referred to are available with synchronized tape commentary from Ahni Productions, Tokyo, and are for sex education of the 13–14 age group.)

The often-recommended unemotional answering of children's questions implies a lack of sensitivity. This is an emotional subject and, in answering questions, regard should be taken for the emotions of the child. Many children meet sex discussion in the open for the first time in schools and are emotionally vulnerable; because of their years of conditioning at home they may feel that nice people do not talk about it. 'Previously teachers felt hesitant to give a straight answer for fear of giving offence at home, yet merely to tell a child to ask mother when he got home doesn't seem right, as the teacher would not answer this way in any other subject.' This comment from the BBC's *School Broadcasting and Sex Education in the Primary School* neatly outlines the dilemma of the teacher needing to be sensitive to the needs of parents, school managers and heads as well as to the needs of the child.

This invasion of personal privacy is the most crucial aspect of sensitivity in sex education, with respect to parents, teachers and children alike. Many parents have gone to some lengths to conceal from their children that they have any sex life at all and when questions are asked, stemming from sex education at school, which break down this carefully-erected barricade, protests are likely to begin. The majority of schools use some method to inform parents about the content and method of sex education courses (see page 37). When approached like this, most parents are only too grateful that the school will provide what they themselves feel unable to.

Teachers often give in to a class's attempt to invade their own personal privacy; frequently classes will push a teacher into saying what intercourse actually feels like for them. Many teachers are embarrassed by this but feel that they must answer the question honestly. But to answer the question by giving one individual's experience is to show lack of awareness of the teacher's position in the continuum of human behaviour; what is good intercourse for him or her may not be satisfactory for the class, and to refer to it may imply a norm which does not exist. Even for the teacher, intercourse will vary in its quality and nature from time to time, so that to imply a norm is not only untrue but can often be a crippling imposition. A simple method of giving the required information used successfully by several teachers is to read the description of sexual intercourse from Desmond Morris's *The Naked Ape* (1967), with due caveats as to the continuum involved and the variation expected by any one individual over a course of time.

Another frequent question to the young or unmarried teacher is as to whether they are virgin or not. Admission in either the negative or the affirmative can be embarrassing, and it is here that the teacher needs to make very clear that his or her private life remains private, unless and until he or she makes the decision that it should be otherwise. Pupils should treat the teacher as they wish to be treated themselves. After all, the teacher does not ask them what

17

they were up to last night, and so is respecting their privacy. Teachers who choose to share their own experiences with their classes must do so with full knowledge of what they are doing; if a young man shares with his class the emotions he felt when his first baby was born, he must still beware of setting up a norm of behaviours which might be unattainable for his class and must clearly show where his experience stands in the continuum of behaviour about human birth. The conditioning of his class and its cultural mores may not be the same as his own.

Finally, in sex education many teachers are not aware of the enormous variation, existing within any one class, of knowledge, attitudes, values and levels of understanding. In any other subject attention would be paid to the need for reinforcement and consolidation, the need for establishing hierarchies of concepts. In sex education instead we have the frequently asked question, 'At what age should a child be told about VD, birth, contraception?' There can be several different levels of teaching, for example about contraception:

First stage. An egg does not necessarily meet a sperm. In primary schools the question usually arises as to why the eggs in the shops don't hatch into chicks, although today it is not uncommon for children under 11 to ask questions about the pill.

Second stage. Methods and means of contraception, e.g. as outlined in Kind and Leedham's programme *Contraception* (1968).

Third stage. Social skills needed to ask for contraceptive advice, how clinics work, cost, selection of the most appropriate method, human variation in response to oral contraceptives. (See Schools Council General Studies Project 16–18, to be published.)

One of the major difficulties in contraceptive education for those in most need of it is in overcoming ideas laid down by early conditioning; at 14 many girls in a South London school were convinced that contraception caused cancer, deformed babies and unsatisfactory sex lives. To change such attitudes is an almost impossible task, and hence the teacher must not only be sensitive to the needs themselves, but to the factors which produced them.

Insight into human behaviour

Insight demands accurate observation based on knowledge of

what to look for; in particular, knowledge is needed by teachers, parents and children, of the physical basis of sexual behaviour. There is still a feeling among educators as expressed in a recent comment in the Times Educational Supplement, 'After all, our impulses to make physical love originate from our brains and are not the monopoly of the biologist'. This demonstrates a lack of awareness of human variation both in the degree of cerebral control which it is possible to exercise and also in the volume of production and size of effects of the sex hormones. In 1965 a group of teachers requested among others a film to be made which would demonstrate 'the *power* of sex. Intelligent girls from good homes . . . have never realized how quickly the point of no return can be reached'. This would now seem to be an international problem, as women become emancipated and allowed into mixed society for the first time with no more education in sexual matters than that deemed necessary for a sheltered home life. One of the many reasons which have forced a demand for sex education is the large numbers of pregnancies among university students in developing countries. 'Sex is a gigantic plot evolved over millions of years to increase the chances of fertilization and reduce the hazards of growth and development' (Dennis Fox, unpublished). This may be a somewhat cynical if not simplistic view, but is certainly more realistic than the idea expressed by the writer in the Times Educational Supplement.

The mechanisms which go to make up this 'gigantic plot'—the physical nature of attraction and pair bonding, the basic drives towards mating and parental care, the effect of hormones on the behaviour particularly of adolescent girls and their often menopausal mothers—figure very infrequently in sex education programmes; this may be because such physical effects are but one factor in determining behaviour and are modified by social, cultural, economic and intellectual influences as well as by the all-pervading concept of human variation. Such inexact ideas demand critical teaching, and perhaps it is not surprising to find teachers avoiding this work from feelings of insecurity about the subject matter. The Nuffield Secondary Science Project has attempted to provide resource material for teachers in this field, and includes Katharina Dalton's excellent book *The Menstrual Cycle* (1970) in its reference list. The relief of anxiety in both girls and boys when the role of the cyclical female hormones in behaviour is discussed is often enormous and leads to a greater intersexual understanding. Few of the lists of questions available showing what adolescents wish to know about sex ever include questions on why a girl feels gloomy or is accident-prone just before menstruation, and few boys ever feel it anything but taboo to ask questions about menstruation. Hence the second of Wilson's criteria is relevant here: being sensitive to the needs of others even when they are not aware of them themselves.

Skills of verbal and social communication

An exhortation frequently bandied about in sex education discussions is 'Give them the facts and let them make up their own minds'. Apart from not recognizing that under the influence of the 'gigantic plot' referred to earlier, the rational making up of minds is difficult, recognition of the part which discussion plays in making decisions is also needed. Adolescents discuss freely with their peer groups, but informal discussion with an informed adult may not be facilitated. There is a classic Swedish film on sex education where children are shown sitting in rigid rows listening to the words of the teacher. This is all too frequently the kind of learning environment set up in this country too, with a bright 'Now, has anyone any questions?' thrown in at the end, which usually produces total silence while the questions go unasked and unanswered.

Local health authority educators are frequently asked to come into classes or youth clubs to lead discussion on sex. Many refuse to begin sex education with any group until they have established a more than superficial communication with the group itself. Good communication between teacher and class is essential if feedback is to be valid and if teaching is to be subordinated to the actual process of learning. It is also essential if vulnerable children are not to be put under emotional strain. To hear a health educator aver that girls had fainted in a VD lesson only because the classroom was poorly ventilated would seem to indicate lack of communication, lack of knowledge of human behaviour and lack of sensitivity to the needs of others.

Communication between members of the class on sexual matters is also important, particularly where culture indicates that for

20

members of the opposite sex to discuss matters is simply not done. Masters and Johnston's second investigation into *Human Sexual Inadequacy* (1970) provides the evidence that it is communication therapy which is needed between partners who can find little satisfaction in their sexual life, not tuition on the athletic and acrobatic aspects of the many positions of intercourse. Uninhibited and freely communicative partners should not be robbed of the joy of discovering the variations possible in intercourse by thoughtless sex education. If they cannot discover it for themselves, then psychiatric and communications therapy is needed, not a digest of the Kama Sutra from the teacher, nor even films showing a rather vitiated and possibly crampingly normative concept of intercourse, as in Martin Cole's film 'Growing Up', among others.

Communication between the sexes, or lack of it, is a considerable factor in the promotion of marital stability, in other fields than in the establishment of satisfactory sexual relations. Discussion between prospective marriage partners of their expected roles in man–woman relationships with respect to family, worksharing, companionship, etc., are essential if disappointment and consequent marital upsets are to be avoided. But perhaps the most important aspect of communication to be fostered in sex education is that between parents and children. Although many countries promote parent education so that the parents may feel more secure in educating their children in sexual matters, it is difficult to see how even a long course of parental education can overcome the conditioning of the previous 20 years. If we are ever to transfer basic sex education from our schools into the hands of the parents, we need to begin with the education of the present generation of school children, so that they may become able and willing to communicate with their own children in years to come. The following extract of an essay seems to indicate that one young man in a Yorkshire school intends to do so. It would be interesting to know if he actually puts his ideas into practice:

I was never told about sex by my parents, mainly because I never asked them anything, I suppose. I soon found out at an early age that when I asked my parents any embarrassing questions, they would tell me to wait a while and ask them later, hoping that I would forget the question. When and if I get married, I intend to tell my offspring the facts of life before they start secondary school, hoping that this will save them a lot of embarrassment at school. If I had been told instead of being left in the dark a lot of agonizing worry would have been spared.

Vocabulary

One of the main difficulties of providing communications skills in sexual matters is that colloquial words are often not used in 'polite' society; doctors, family planning clinics and those involved in any medical work concerned with sex organs often find patients are unable to describe their troubles, as they have little knowledge of the respectable/acceptable terms. Why should not patients be encouraged to use the vernacular? For one reason many are unwilling to do so, as it causes them embarrassment, and for another, no part of the English language is so rich in creative synonyms as those words used in talking about human reproduction. At least the medical words have common currency, not only in this country but to a large extent throughout the world—an important point in a mobile society. Secondly, it would be an impossible task to remove the shock power of many colloquialisms in common usage. Cyril Bibby used to recommend to his students as an antidote to classes giggling in sex education, that the teacher list all known 'dirty' words on the board, and then translate them into acceptable terms. The fact that the teacher actually knew of the existence of such words usually provoked a roar of laughter from the class; that he was not shocked by them reduced the potential for whispered comments which provoked the sniggers. Having indicated that sex was a proper thing to discuss with a responsible adult, the climate of discussion was thereby raised to a more mature level. Teachers should, however, be cautious of using methods like this which are appropriate to a certain sort of personality which may be unlike their own. Some in America have lost their jobs for using this technique.

The possession of the appropriate vocabulary is one thing, the social ability to use it is another. Many adults have the necessary knowledge about contraception but are unable to take action on it as they are prevented by lack of social skills from attending a Family Planning clinic. How will they tell their boss they need time off to attend in clinic hours? What if someone they know sees them at the clinic? How can they ask that giggly girl in the chemist's for what they want? Some even need to be taught how to use a telephone to find out clinic hours in a new part of the country. Social skills are an essential part of any sex education programme, even if this only involves familiarizing adolescents with clinic and hospital procedures.

These are only some of the major aspects of communication in the field of sex education—a whole book could be written on communications problems and methods alone. Later sections of this book on the mass media (page 63) and the provision of the extra parental counsellor (page 74) will deal more pragmatically with other important aspects.

Making judgements of right and wrong for the individual and for society

'What was good enough for my father was good enough for me. I didn't have any sex education when I was young and it did me no harm.' 'I didn't have any sexual intercourse until I was 25, why should today's young people expect to have it any earlier?' Unfortunately, the rapid changes in the structure of society in recent years show no signs of slowing down, and a changing society means changing needs; this is one of the basic causes of the generation gap in communication. It might be sensible to try to list the changes which have taken place in the lifetime of the present generation of parents, and use this as a basis for discussion with the opponents of sex education, although, as mentioned previously, rational discussion is likely to have little effect on the attitudes, prejudices and value judgements which have resulted from many years' conditioning.

But sex education needs to provide for the young at least some of the skills in thinking and applying moral principles to individual situations rather than imposing a moral code which has to be applied to any situation, however inappropriate. The latter, of course, is much easier—a rigid set of rules, which needs little thought, is what many people seek, and what many others find hard to relinquish. Student teachers in a sex education course pressed the lecturer to say what answer they should give when a pupil asks whether pre-marital intercourse is right or wrong. The lecturer replied that it was first wise to ask why the question had been asked and secondly whether the teacher knew enough about the background, attitudes and culture of the questioner and his society to be able to give a useful answer. The students replied that this had not answered their question—was the answer yes or no? This shows that it is not only the unintelligent or intellectually inadequate who seek black and white answers when the true reply comes only in varying shades of grey.

Giving adolescents skills and information to decide what is right or wrong for the individual is difficult enough. Helping them to make the right decisions for society and the world as a whole is even more difficult, as the full factual knowledge of the situation may not be available and considerable powers of abstract thought are needed to project the result of an individual act into international proportions. It may be easy for a middle class Englishman to see the benefits for his own standard of living and that of the population in general if he limits his family, but for a Bengali farmer accustomed to thinking that he needs to produce a large number of children so that at least some may survive to look after him in old age, it is difficult to realize that less children will mean better medical care and hence more are likely to survive, or that his present rate of reproduction will mean that the available food supplies are insufficient for all.

So this aspect of sex education rests on good general education and a considerable ability to see the future consequences of present action. Bernstein's work as applied by Lawton (1968) would indicate that there is a large sub-culture in this country where such pre-requisites cannot be assumed; there are people in England today who still believe that another child will not really matter as there will be another family allowance to collect, without realizing that the expense of rearing a child is far greater than the expected extra income.

Finally, the failure of sex education to provide means whereby decisions can be made by adolescents other than at the moment of crisis is being overcome in many schools by the use of decision-making material provided, for example, by the Schools Council Humanities Curriculum Project, the Schools Council General Studies Project, the Nuffield Science Project and the Schools Council

Moral Education Project. Evaluation of attitude changes is being undertaken by the Humanities Curriculum Project which has already run a battery of 21 tests and instruments on a pre-test basis. Results from post-testing will be available in 1972.

The ability to do what is right

Man is not a wholly rational animal and much of sexual behaviour is not due to rational decisions. Rational decisions may in fact be made, but the individual may be unable to carry them out because of the influence of many factors, not least the powers of physical attraction. It is doubtful whether any girl under sixteen rationally desires a baby, and yet the pregnancy rate for this group rises yearly. The lack of a secure self-image and hence a yielding to peer group pressures may be one factor. Certainly a lack of knowledge of the power of physical attraction may be another. It is doubtful whether sex education can be useful here, as the underlying causes are psychological and social as well as physiological, and the concepts involved too abstract for those most in need of them. A very experienced London headmistress commented that for the 14-year-old girl who wants a baby 'because it would be something of my own', for girls who get pregnant hoping that at least they will get some attention from the welfare officer, even if their boy doesn't marry them, the basic problem is that the child in question may well have been unwanted herself and has certainly been brought up by parents unaware of the needs of children for understanding communication and genuine friendship. What is needed here is to break the vicious circle of the unwanted child poorly cared for in mental and emotional health (although often physically healthy and materially well provided for) who tends to produce unwanted children in turn. Jane Madders of the City of Birmingham College of Education is perhaps the foremost in this field. She introduces such girls into playgroups as working helpers, so that they learn by experience and by contact with experts of the child's needs for mental and emotional development; incidentally, the girls also improve their reading skills in a way which does not involve loss of face, by reading simple stories to the playgroup, and many of them go home with the mothers of the children to see how the child behaves in a home environment. Thus skills which the middle classes learn by imitation or improvement of parental roles and constant reference to books are gained through experience by girls who are unlikely to acquire them in any other way.

The more one examines sex education, the more complex it is seen to be. The idea that illegitimate pregnancies may be prevented by playgroup work is only one example of the devious lines of thought which must be followed if we are to deal with irrationally based sex behaviour, and treat the underlying disease rather than dealing superficially with its symptoms.

Psychological freedom

It is possible that people do exist who are completely free from psychological blockages about all aspects of sex education; if this is so, then they must be rare. On the other hand, to others nothing is ever half so immoral as sex.

While at one end of the continuum of human behaviour there are those who make a lifetime's hobby of crying 'filth' to all sex education and at the other those who think nothing is too sacred to be divulged, most teachers will find themselves in the middle with one or two minor embarrassments about various aspects of sex. Warren Johnson in his excellent book *Human Sexual Behaviour and Sex Education* (1968) quotes, 'the case of a superintendent of schools of a medium-sized city who actively blocked sex education—not, as he insisted to his board and himself, for moral reasons—but because, as he suddenly confided, he resented his own impotency so profoundly'. A large number of the younger generation suspect that similar reasons of sexual frustration lie behind the thinking of many who are so vocal in seeking to suppress sex education. Perhaps one of the most important aspects of the subject which is dealt with in no programme to my knowledge is that which concerns the inadvisability of clinging on to a waning sex drive in later life, and of making such behaviour unnecessary by the provision of other reasons for intercourse between the sexes apart from sexual intercourse. The middle-aged divorced or separated wife advertising in the newspaper columns for a mate always stresses that she is still physically attractive—presumably those who are no longer nubile weep silently and don't advertise. The American senior citizens are perhaps the most obvious example of the fruitless chase after youthful physical attraction and it is pathetic to read that sex shops in this country (the modern equivalent of the purveyors of love philtres in mediaeval times) are patronized mostly by the 40-plus age group, with a majority of customers over 50, as are strip-clubs.

For the teacher at the centre of the continuum, however, there is a necessity to discover his or her own psychological imbalance, in private rather than in front of the class. There are many teachers who honestly admit that they are unfitted to teach sex education and one must admire them for making such statements; those who are pushed unwillingly into work about which they feel embarrassed, guilty or ashamed can do little good to themselves or their pupils. Others feel inadequate in certain fields. For example, a woman who has been unable to have children may recognize that she is emotionally jealous of girls who produce unwanted babies with ease, and that her attitude to teaching about this aspect may well suffer from a desire to lean over backwards to be fair to such girls rather than to censure them. Similarly, a man who has perhaps been punished for masturbating when young may hand this aspect of the work over to a colleague who he feels might treat the subject more objectively. Children, too, can lose their psychological freedom about sexual matters; the lifting of the heavy load of unwarranted anxiety which many carry is a prime objective of sex education.

The use of Wilson's criteria as an analytical tool

While philosophers may carp at this simplification of Wilson's work, teachers have found it of use in sorting out their ideas on sex education. The following table gives some indication of how it can be used. Readers may like to amplify the notes shown here or use this table with respect to particular aspects of sex education such as contraception, or the means of establishing a secure self-image in sexual matters for adolescent boys.

It has been said that Wilson's criteria are not ideologically neutral. It is difficult to see how they could be, but it is certain that they are neutral enough to have been received by all denominations of Christianity and by Muslims, Hindus and Buddhists on courses in the UK, as a most valuable basis for thinking constructively about morals and sex education. Their use in the identification of overall objectives clarifies the problems of selecting short-term pragmatic objectives and methods for different ages and cultural groups. Once one has considered the objectives of sex education with reference to Wilson's criteria, it becomes obvious that thinking in this field had previously been superficial, confused and directionless.

Criteria for moral education used to help analysis of problems of introducing sex education

Criteria for moral education	*Educators*
Those who are morally educated take *equal concern* for the needs of others as they do for themselves.	Must think out fully WHY sex education is deemed necessary and avoid busybodying do-goodism.
To be able to take equal concern, they must be *sensitive and perceptive* of the needs of others.	Often not sensitive to variations in human knowledge, attitudes, levels of understanding which may exist in one seemingly homogeneous class.
To be sensitive and perceptive they need *insight* into human behaviour and knowledge of what lies behind it.	Few teachers are aware of the physical basis of behaviour or of man's basic needs and drives.
Sensitivity, insight and equal concern are of little use if they cannot be communicated; *skills of both verbal and social communication* are needed.	Lack of communication is often due to an insecure self-image. Embarrassed teachers are worse than none at all?
If all these other criteria are fulfilled people should be able to make *judgements of right and wrong, not only for themselves but for society as a whole*.	This needs education—the long-term aim of many societies is population reduction—but this is difficult for individuals to appreciate. Short-term aims are commonest where education in abstract thought is least.
Having done all this, are people able to *do what they think is right?*	Teachers must be aware of and systematically tackle the peer group pressures against this.
To put all this into action people need to be *psychologically free*—or at least to be aware of the handicaps left to them by previous experience.	Teachers should not be pressurized to teach any part of the work about which they feel emotionally disturbed. They should be encouraged to become aware of their handicaps.

Criteria for moral education used to help analysis of problems of introducing sex education

Parents	Children
May not realize full extent of child's needs in changing society.	Do not take equal concern for each other. Early and late developers are often teased unmercifully. Boys and girls are not aware of each other's needs.
Own desire for personal privacy may overcome sensitivity to child's needs. Parents may not want children to think of them as sexual animals.	They need to be sensitive to their parents' needs too.
Few begin child rearing with any knowledge of child's mental and physical development—should they continue to learn as they go along, perhaps at the expense of the children?	It is often therapeutic for children to learn the basis of their own behaviour. For example, girls are relieved to know that their moodiness is in some part due to hormonal fluctuations rather than madness.
Lack of communication between parents may lead to marital breakdown. Certainly leads to rebellious adolescents.	Children need to learn the appropriate and accepted vocabulary, but they also seek security of self-image during adolescence and may be too shy to use the words.
What was good enough for my father is good enough for my children—only as long as the structure of society remains the same.	Children should not have to judge for themselves with too few facts in a moment of crisis. They need practice in expressing value judgements on sexual behaviour problems, before they become involved themselves.
The special relationship of the parent may preclude adolescents taking their advice and support. The extra-parental counsellor's advice is more effective here.	Even knowing about contraceptives, knowing where and at what time to get them—are young brides not often too embarrassed to do anything about it?

Criteria for moral education used to help analysis of problems of introducing sex education

Parents	Children
Many do not accept that curiosity about one's own body is natural.	Freedom from guilt and shame are a primary objective in sex education. Children WANT to do the right thing—so good sex education can aid their psychological freedom.

Possible action to be taken

Teachers need more than superficial knowledge of the attitudes and values of their classes before choosing an appropriate course.

Any sex education programme must be introduced gradually and respect the personal privacy of parents, teachers and children alike.

The basic concept of human variation in behaviour must be established, as well as human variation in growth.
Nuffield Secondary Science work on adolescent growth spurts, effect of hormones. Heinemann Individual Learning Project on puberty.

Teenagers often use the imparting of sexual knowledge to gain respect and admiration from friends, often developing a climate of discussion which implies that sex is dirty. 'Clean' discussion using proper words needed.

Cultural differences due to changing society producing a generation gap. Structured discussion of problems by film, newspaper agony columns, Alan Harris Questions about Living. Can only be based on a high level of general education.

In any course, much can be taught to large groups and yet action may depend on individual counselling either from parent, teacher, trained counsellor but usually from peer group.

Can guilt-prone teachers produce guilt-free children?

References

BRITISH BROADCASTING CORPORATION (1971). *School Broadcasting and Sex Education in the Primary School*, from 35, Marylebone High Street, London, W1M 4AA.

DALTON, K. (1970). *The Menstrual Cycle*. London: Penguin.

GREEN, L. (1970). 'Identifying and overcoming barriers to the diffusion of knowledge about family planning.' *Advances in Fertility Control*, **5**, 2, reprinted in *J. Inst. Health Educ.* (1971), **9**, 1.

JOHNSON, W. (1968). *Human Sexual Behaviour and Sex Education* (2nd edn.). Philadelphia: Lea & Febiger.

KIND, R. W. and LEEDHAM, J. (1968). *Contraception*. Programmed Sex Information Series. London: Longmans.

LAWTON, D. (1968). *Social Class, Language and Education*. London: Routledge & Kegan Paul.

LONDON COUNTY COUNCIL (1964). *Some Notes on Sex Education*. Now out of print.

MASTERS, W. H. and JOHNSON, V. E. (1970). *Human Sexual Inadequacy*. London: Churchill.

MORRIS, D. (1967). *The Naked Ape*. London: Galaxy.

NUFFIELD SECONDARY SCIENCE (1971). *Theme 3—The Biology of Man*. London: Longmans.

RADELFINGER, S. (1965). 'Some effects of fear-rousing communications on preventive health behaviour.' *Health Education Monographs*, **19**, 1–16. Society of Public Health Educators (USA).

REID, D. and BOOTH, P. (1970). *How Life Begins*. London: Heinemann.

SCHOOLS COUNCIL GENERAL STUDIES PROJECT. (To be published in 1972.) Inquiries should be made to The Secretary, General Studies Project, The King's Manor, York.

SCHOOLS COUNCIL MORAL EDUCATION PROJECT (1972). *Lifeline*. London: Longmans.

WILSON, J. (1965). *Logic and Sexual Morality*. London: Penguin.

WILSON, J. (1970). *Moral Thinking*. London: Heinemann.

YOUNG, M. (1967). 'Review of research and studies related to health education: methods and materials.' *Health Education Monographs*, **25**, 8–24. USA: Society of Public Health Educators.

Teaching Aids

SCHOOLS COUNCIL HUMANITIES PROJECT (1970). 'Relations Between the Sexes.' 'The Family.' Teachers' Kits. London: Heinemann. £10 each.

SOCIETY OF EDUCATIONAL RESEARCH FOR SEX PROBLEMS. 'Hello! Thirteen.' Ahni Production Ltd., 4–3–8 Kamiyoga, Setagaya, Tokyo, Japan. Set of slides with synchronized tape commentary. About £40.

CHAPTER TWO

Sex Education at Different Ages; at Home, School and Youth Club

Infant and pre-school sex education

IT IS IN THE HOME that a child absorbs attitudes towards the body and its functions, ideas about taboos, and feelings of acceptance or rejection and about his physical nature long before his mind is capable of taking in facts by anything other than non-verbal communication. The puzzlement or even shock which many children experience when they first meet the dirty joke, often at school, and a totally different interpretation of bodily functions from that which they have been used to, is something which needs parental support in the highest degree.

It is often because parents are afraid of 'What he'll come out with in front of other people' that they hesitate to give sex information to their children; it is understandable but sad that the *faux pas* made by children only half-aware of social taboos, which are themselves questionable, should militate against the transmission of necessary knowledge. It is felt by many people that a parent loses a valuable dimension in his relationship with his child if open communication on sexual matters at an early age is not possible. If a child is upset by obscenity at school, or is subject to experiment by the sexually curious children met at school, not to be able to go home and get reassurance and support is tragic; having to keep such matters to himself in secrecy and shame is hardly helpful to the processes of growing up.

Attitudes which are set at this early age are very difficult to overcome in later life. Many countries begin their sex education at 13 or 14, when much of it will be too little and too late for a large number of children. It is in pre-puberty that a child can make most use of parental communication on sex. After puberty matters become complicated by the adolescent rebellion against parents, the generation gap, the search for a secure self-image and the influence of the peer group; at the time, the parent is too often the last person to whom an adolescent will go for help and discussion, hence the need for an extra-parental counsellor, as Derek Miller puts it (see page 76).

There are innumerable variations in the willingness of parents to answer their pre-school child's questions on sex and bodily functions —some parents can be too keen! One six-year-old girl came to her father who was working in the garden and asked him 'What's sex?' He, conscientiously, did his parental duty at great length, only stopping when he saw the growing bewilderment of his child. 'Why did you ask?' 'Because Mummy says tea will be ready in a couple of secs.' It is always difficult to tread the middle way in any field, and especially in sex education. It is probably useful to remember that while a parent feels that a full explanation must be given, often the child is not capable of assimilating it, and would prefer a short simplification, coming back to ask for further extension when he has time to think around the answer.

One of the most useful books for parents to use with their children at the pre-school and infant stage in answering questions about sex is the Time-Life publication *How Babies are Made* (Andrey and Schepp, 1969); the large, bright pictures, if a trifle coy and cosy to British eyes, are attractive, explanatory and provide a useful visual peg on which to hang a large number of words. Marie Neurath's books provide similar gay, simple explanations for an older age group. The Time-Life book can also be obtained as a film strip with explanatory notes for parents on how to explain complex concepts with simplicity, although it rather euphemistically skirts around intercourse. This brings up an important point; we seem to get ourselves into a position where we feel a sense of failure if we don't make even the most complex relationships simple and understandable to the child asking the questions. 'You won't understand it until you're older' has often been an excuse for not giving information on sex because of embarrassment and with the swing of the pendulum too few people realize how true it is still today.

How can one explain the emotions of a sexual relationship to a young child? It is of course impossible and this should be admitted, while asking the child if he can describe exactly what he feels like on Christmas morning, or when he hugs the cat or his puppy. Some things are indescribable by all except poets and literary geniuses and we lesser mortals should admit defeat.

B

To leave young children vulnerable to the impact of sex information from adverts, television and prurient school friends is indefensible; reports frequently made by Dr. Eickhoff, the Birmingham psychiatrist, that children are emotionally shocked by sex education in schools are quite true. But one must ask why these children were left in such a vulnerable position not only to sex information in school, but also to the many sources of worry and anxiety out of school too; there is no excuse for ignoring the fact that unless *all* sex information is suppressed from *every* source, unprepared children are going to react emotionally to it.

It would seem reasonable for parents of children who distress others with their obscenities (particularly boys who attempt to remove little girls' knickers, or who follow them home from school with frightening innuendo, if not direct assault) to be censored by society for failing in their duty to other children as well as to their own. This concept is rarely mentioned in public debate possibly because of a lack of communication of the disturbed children with their parents.

Sex education in the primary school

'With regard to sex education many teachers evade their responsibility. They are reluctant to become involved in such an emotive subject. It is a reluctance tinged with fear of possible consequences to themselves or their career, and they fall back upon the fallacious argument that parents are the ideal people to do it. They delude themselves that parenthood automatically confers some magical quality of intuition and knowledge concerning every aspect of a child's development. This is patently not so.' This view was put forward by Albert Chanter, one of the foremost experts in primary school sex education, in a study day for teachers held by the National Childbirth Trust in 1970. Nevertheless, Chanter is very much aware of the danger of usurping a parent's rights and feelings in this matter and takes careful and well-thought-out action to ensure that the school complements the parental influence and enhances it rather than merely promoting a take-over (see page 37).

An ever-growing number of primary schools work on the family grouping, integrated day approach, and in such conditions sex education takes place informally, children's questions being answered as they arise, projects developing from them on animal rearing, class heights and weights and individual work explained to children by children. This does not mean that formal teaching is totally absent; a school, undergoing trials of a discovery and investigation project, after the initial impetus of joy in doing something different, were faced with a moan from the children, 'Why doesn't someone just *tell* us something for a change?' Telling a story with pictures about birth, seeing a film about how the chicken gets into the egg, about parental care in animals, are also part of sex education in the informal primary school.

More important than the transmission of facts is the provision of a climate of communication where children feel happy to ask questions and where a worried child can find supportive counselling from a reassuring adult. The awareness that facts must be seen in a relevant framework of human relationships is apparent in the scheme of work for primary schools produced by Albert Chanter (1966) and Exeter Education Committee (1970). In Phoenix, Arizona, a parent complained about school sex education because her 12-year-old son practised what he had learned about intercourse on his four-year-old sister; the school may well have been at fault here in not placing facts in the context of the considerate way of life, but it is possible that the parents were not entirely guiltless.

Another danger in primary school sex education is that too much insensitive work with animals may lead to the concept of man as just another animal rather than a very special case of an animal with a brain and emotions. To give a *reductio ad absurdum* of what might happen, a doctor (private communication) reported that the couple had come to him for fertility treatment, in a rural area; on investigation he found that they only had intercourse twice yearly because that is what happened in the farm animals! (This was 15 years ago, before intensive farming methods had reached this particular community.) It is always dangerous to transfer conclusions from animal behaviour directly to human behaviour, whether in matters of aggression as exemplified by the Ardrey school of thought (Ashley Montagu, 1968) or in sexual activities. What is 'natural' is often dubiously accurate and may have little relevance to today's structure of society.

'I walked the three miles home from school convinced that I was bleeding to death', said a Durham schoolgirl in 1910, 'but when I told my mother she just laughed and said it happens to everyone. I resolved there and then that any children I ever had would be told about menstruation long before it happened.' It seems unbelievable that there are still some parents today who leave their girls uninformed about menstruation, except from what they can pick up from friends or surreptitious reading of women's magazines and books. Apart from the lack of basic factual information itself, its omission implies that such matters are not proper for discussion, and that secrecy should attend the experience of menstruation. Girls need to know more than the basic facts—'What will I do if it happens first at school? Everyone will know if it stains my dress.' This is a common worry. With earlier maturity more and more girls experience the menarche in primary school and many schools are indeed providing the information necessary. But relatively few are helping these girls over the emotional and social problems that beginning menstruation raises, especially in the way of giving such education to boys as well, so that the embarrassment caused by the unfulfilled curiosity of boys in the class is minimized. The considerate way of life for both sexes in early adolescence is fostered if girls are informed that boys have their own problems of unexpected erections and wet dreams, which do not adhere to a regular timetable as menstruation does. Fifty years ago pregnancy was something which women were secretive about, while few are ashamed of pregnancy today; it would seem reasonable to consider menstruation in a similar light.

The total picture of sex education in the primary school depends on the concept of freedom of the curriculum in British education—freedom for apathy as well as for excellence and sensitivity. One cannot assume a that child changing schools at 11 has had any sex education at all. Don Reid and Phil Booth of Thomas Bennett School, Crawley (1970), have developed a programmed learning approach to ensure, amongst other objectives, that all the first-year pupils have a certain amount of basic knowledge. The Nuffield Secondary Science Project (1967) found that in their trial schools, even 13-year-olds were lacking in basic terminology and facts. These had to be inserted into their course. However, with the widespread use of the Combined Science Projects work in the 11–13 range, and the impact of the BBC Merry-go-round and radio-vision programmes on the younger age groups, the position has improved, although it is known that many schools still give no sex education at all, before puberty, for a variety of reasons.

Methods of informing parents

'My first reaction was one of indignation that anyone should suggest I cannot instruct my own child, but I realize that there are some who wouldn't. Some say it is too young, but I do not agree.' This quotation from Chanter (1968) indicates a reasonable and prevalent attitude of parents when consulted about the introduction of sex education into a primary school. Chanter, in common with most teachers in a similar situation, had consulted the parents and given them full information on the proposed course by means of an introductory letter inviting them to meet and discuss the situation. Chanter's description of the variety of parental reactions is well worth reading and it is interesting to compare the 100 per cent contact and agreement he reached in a localized situation, where his own personality played a large part in establishing communication, with the problems facing both BBC and ITV when introducing sex education programmes to a much larger and more anonymous audience. Larger schools in urban areas would also find more difficulties than Chanter; keen and middle class parents will come to discussions, but those parents perhaps in most need of them often do not.

Twenty years ago in what was then an LCC grammar school, basic sex instruction was given to the first-year girls, including simple, well-illustrated books on birth, menstruation, etc. These books were sent home with a note to parents before the course began. Few children were ever withdrawn from the classes and most parental comment expressed relief and delight that the school was undertaking this work; many wished that they had had such books themselves in adolescence.

In contrast, in another London school in 1970, in an area with a large proportion of immigrants (Carribbean, Hindu and Muslim), letters were sent to parents explaining the course and offering withdrawal. To the surprise of the staff, no withdrawals were requested; it was, however, suspected that this did not indicate that

37

the local imam had given his approval, rather that half the letters never reached the parents, some were not read, and others, if read, were not comprehended.

A health education adviser who has held meetings with hundreds of parents in one area over the years had only three opponents of his courses. In addition, he found that parents would come up to him privately at the end of such meetings and discuss other family problems connected with sex. Finally he found that the courses had become part of the accepted pattern and that after a few years of parents' meetings, the need for them to be held at all disappeared.

Not all parents' meetings go so smoothly; in 1970 a group of middle class parents in Surrey refused to sanction the showing of a film on birth (acceptable and successful in many similar schools) to their daughters, while in East London, both parents and teachers rejected the BBC radiovision visuals, which they felt were 'dirty pictures'. (The two radiovision programmes consist of a film strip and a synchronized tape commentary, for eight- to nine-year-olds, with music and deal very simply with pregnancy, birth and intercourse in the programme 'Where Do Babies Come From?' and with changes in adolescence in 'Growing Up', which also includes menstruation.)

What factors does Chanter's small-scale and very personal exercise have in common with the problems of contacting large numbers of parents which faced the BBC on the introduction of its radiovision and Merry-go-round programmes? (These were three television films on 'Beginning' which dealt with gestation, 'Birth' and 'Full Circle' showing fertilization.) The Merry-go-round series is intended for seven- to nine-year-olds, but the audience for its sex education programmes extended from seven to eleven.

1. *The decision that parents must be consulted.* How very different from the old idea of the fifth-form talk (see page 9); if parents had been consulted about this, one wonders how many would have agreed to its form and content. It must also be recorded that in one London school in 1971, while both parents and teachers were in agreement about the proposed course for primary children, their wishes were vetoed by the school managers.

2. *The organization required to do so.* Chanter's problems here were relatively small, while the BBC had to devote a great deal of

38

thought to the subject and succeeded admirably. Their report (BBC, 1971) shows that for the radiovision programmes 83 per cent of the schools were able to achieve and arrange meetings with parents and in most of these the film strips and tapes were shown. The remaining schools either informed the parents by letter, advised them to see the showings of the programmes, especially for parents and teachers on national TV, or, in schools where sex education was already well-established, the heads merely expressed their intentions of showing the filmstrips.

With the Merry-go-round programmes, however, the difficulty or possibly (although this was not mentioned in the report) the expense of obtaining the films (which at the time were not available for hiring) meant that few heads showed them to parents, although parents were informed of the late night showings on TV as for radiovision. Those who already had a sex education programme took these films as part of the Merry-go-round series and did not make any special case for them; they were proved right, there were indeed no adverse comments from parents.

3. *The right of parents to withdraw children.* Chanter had only a few withdrawals and he wrote to these pointing out the isolation which would thereby be caused to their children. None of these parents then renewed their objections. This was paralleled by the BBC experience; agreement was at least 90 per cent and many who first objected later changed their minds. In the Grampian TV showing of their Living and Growing series (see page 103) parents who had been doubtful in 1968 were quite confident about the programmes in 1970, but there were actually more withdrawals.

4. *Appreciation of such meetings.* Both Chanter and the BBC were mindful of the need for both parents to be able to attend meetings and arranged times accordingly, e.g. the BBC reported that the radiovision meetings had resulted in closer relationships between parents and teachers in this field and it is implicit also in their evidence that the relationship between parent and child became more communicative after such meetings. Chanter reports that after one of his meetings a parent asked what one did with the child who does not ask questions.

The above may paint too rosy a picture; of the 11,000 schools using Merry-go-round, 77 per cent did not take the programmes on

Figures about informing parents from the Grampian TV showings of 'Living and Growing' in 1968 and 1970

	1968	1970
Schools sent letters informing parents	68%	71%
Asked parents' permission	'A few'	38%
Discussion with parents	14%	17%
Discussion not needed, parents' views already known	—	9%
Number of parents who viewed the programme	'Many'	50%
Parents' comments	Favourable, 46%	'Largely favourable'
	Unfavourable, one letter to Grampian	Gratitude and relief predominant
Pupils withdrawn by parents	4 in 1 school 2 girls from menstruation programme.	40 from 23 schools

Parents who had been doubtful before, were quite confident in 1970.

sex education. This was due to a variety of factors which included the hostility of the parents, division of opinion on the staffroom, and the feelings of some heads that it would be foolish to swim against the tide of local public opinion. Society in the United Kingdom is not only multi-racial, including Ukrainians as well as Kenyan Asians, but has a multiplicity of small subcultures whose opinions must be respected when introducing education on this emotional subject.

Sex education in secondary schools

There used to be a wide difference between selective, academic schools and non-selective, secondary modern schools with respect to sex education; on the whole the grammar schools tended to limit it, particularly in the case of boys, to give the basic biological facts and perhaps a little moralizing at most, whereas teachers of less academic classes have been more aware of the urgent needs of pupils who may marry shortly after they leave school. As Stenhouse says in the introduction to the Teacher's Handbook on *Relations*

40

Between the Sexes (Schools Council Humanities Project, 1970), 'Pupils of 14 and over generally are, and most certainly ought to be, interested in relations between the sexes. Sixteen is in our society the legal age of consent. Many pupils who leave school at 16 will already be looking towards marriage. Virtually all will already have had sexual experience of some sort and some will have had intercourse. There is no controversial area which more urgently asks for understanding on the part of the pupils.' Contrast this with the attitude of the academic schools which may be summed up by the Nuffield 'O' level Biology approach in Year 1, i.e. to 11-year-olds. 'The subject of sexual reproduction is *always a difficult one to teach*, especially where it involves man himself. Following the reproductive processes in other mammals, human reproduction presented, *as it should be* in a purely factual manner, will be accepted in the same vein.' Later in the Teacher's Guide comes the classic and much quoted statement under the heading 'The birth of a baby': 'It is not possible to anticipate the many questions which this section may provide, but there may be opportunity for making comparisons between human birth and the birth of domestic or farm animals with which some of the children may be familiar.'

However, it is all too easy to mock these pioneers of 1963, working in a quite different, if less heated, climate of discussion about the subject than we are today. The rewriting of Nuffield 'O' level, taking into account teachers' comments and today's attitudes is taking place at the moment. One part of the work which had clearly set out objectives and which has stood the test of time is the section on chick embryology, where the remarkable organization of a relatively structureless yolk into the blood, bones, nerves and feathers of a living chick is well set out. Even here, however, the sensitivities of the class and often those of the teacher to the killing of a living organism provoked a lively exchange of letters in the Times Educational Supplement (Limburd, Brogden, 5.4.68). It is for this reason that the Nuffield Secondary Science Project has produced two film loops showing the development of the chick, so that teachers who prefer may use them instead of the live animals. This is the kind of thing which can happen when factual objectives are treated in isolation from the objectives of moral education.

There have always been a few secondary schools where the head

41

or the Chaplain has worked closely with the Biology department and perhaps the English and PE specialists also to provide a well-integrated course on sex education. Today with such a vast amount of material from various curriculum reform projects, both national and local, there is a strong case for a co-ordinator who could spend most of his time just becoming familiar with the mass of material in the Humanities, Moral Education and Nuffield Secondary Science projects and producing a synthesis of all three best suited to his own school. A boy's grammar school in the Midlands has in fact done just this, not only for sex education but also dealing with addiction and problems of adjusting to adult life. The master concerned has a working party representing all shades of opinion, and one lightly timetabled year in which to examine and synthesize resource material for a course to be followed by form masters of boys of 14–18 with outside specialists' help and counselling.

The Humanities Curriculum Project—Schools Council

The project has two sets of material particularly relevant to sex education: 'Relations between the Sexes' and 'The Family'. But the other resources kits on war, education, poverty, living in cities, people and work, law and order and race relations also inquire into a variety of sexual matters.

On first looking at these resources, all one can say is here's richness. Few teachers or, for that matter, few average and above average school children could resist becoming totally immersed in these collections of cartoons, first class writing, photographs of today and yesterday. They take the form of a pile of sheets which invites total disorganization but does not give that awful feeling of 'Heavens, I must slog through all this' which a textbook of similar dimensions would do. Nor, therefore, does it impose rigidity on the teacher but leaves him free to select or reject. There are also tapes of interviews, of folksongs, of poetry reading and seductive lists of recommended films; it is always advisable for teachers to see films before they can be sure of their suitability for a class and also to enable them to structure the work around the film so that viewing does not become a passive, sleep-inducing process. Teachers of the Humanities project, however, will need strong moral fibre to ensure that they do not convince themselves that it is essential to devote time to seeing *all* the films recommended in 'Relations between the Sexes'. Some 90 viewing hours in all are required. The range is from 'A Victorian lady in her boudoir', to a 'Deadpan study of Hugh Hefner', and his Bunny Club ethos. These are in the 'Relations between the Sexes' kit which deals with male–female roles, how the sexes meet and judge each other, courtship, marriage from the point of view of the unmarried (marriage situations are dealt with brilliantly in the kit on 'The Family'), as well as work on the unmarried themselves. Nonconformity in sexual patterns, controls on inter-sexual relationships, generation gaps, love as opposed to romance and sex, prudence and morality, also feature in the material. Lawrence Stenhouse, the Director of the project, states clearly in the introduction to the work that 'It is superficial and educationally undesirable to regard this as an ethical supermarket from which one chooses a view. This being so, it is highly undesirable to use evidence on sex and morality early in the inquiry. The "answers" are not there. The function of the evidence is to show the range of moral positions held.'

This idea of neutrality is a fundamental philosophy of the project. 'Neutrality means that the teacher should not propagate his own view but be prepared to see the pupils treat all views according to consistent critical principles', said Stenhouse in an introduction to the project (New Society, 24 July, 1969). Too often the teacher uses leading questions to turn an open discussion into a guessing game where the class tries to find the answers which gain most approval from sir. Total neutrality is impossible, as a teacher can show bias by his selection of the resource material itself. Indeed there are times when a teacher needs consciously to nail his colours to the mast, as pupils may become frustrated by his permanent fence sitting. However, this kind of exercise of disciplined criticism and discussion makes one feel, when it is seen in action, that democracy might actually become a working reality rather than a nebulous ideal. Stenhouse is currently carrying out a long-term survey of the attitude shifts and the effects of the total impact of the project and has just completed the pre-testing; final results will be available in 1972. Is it too much to hope that by the use of such methods we might expect a higher standard of debate, both public and Parliamentarian, in the future?

Apart from the education in forming opinions which this project stimulates, here also is an encouragement to read, and to write creatively; Adrian Henri's poem 'Love is . . .' encouraged one class of not very verbal 14-year-olds in an immigrant area to write a startling set of poems on the same lines. They showed a fair appreciation of the difference between Eros and Agape, as well as a number of cultural and personal views, all of which were discussed by the rest of the class. Skills of non-verbal communication are also fostered in the interpretation of photographs ranging from a determinedly jolly set of rugger players singing their determinedly dirty songs in the communal shower to a pregnant, roller-wearing mum in a supermarket; this was 'Included as showing the treble role of wife (the curlers so her hair will be well done in the evening), child bearer and housekeeper. Is it fair to say that there is also a sense of the worry of budgeting and deciding what to buy?'

So much for the material on 'Relations between the sexes'; it is complemented by similarly structured resources on 'The Family'. This is particularly welcome, as it gives a really wide view of marriage as it is lived and not as it is imagined in the fantasies of the human mind of the fiction of women novelists. One of the more positive objectives of sex education is education for marriage. This all too often consists of a few exhortatory remarks about relationships and a lot about budgeting and marriage etiquette; Stenhouse's material should be made required reading for all school leavers. It ranges from Vanessa Redgrave to St. Paul, and across several cultures; it even includes Leon Rosselson's 'Invisible married breakfast blues'. Apart from giving insight into a wide variety of relationships within marriage, sections of the material should indicate to those in haste to marry when young that marriage often produces more problems than it solves. Much education about marriage leaves the adolescent still out of touch with reality and probability. He feels that others may fail, but that he will succeed, and while one would not wish to douse the flame of human optimism, awareness of the enormous number of factors involved in a satisfying marital relationship cannot but be gained by the study of this material.

Criticism has been made that it is too difficult for the users of a restricted code of speech, and for the poor readers; this problem could be overcome in many ways, such as reading it to the poor readers, simplifying it for those to whom the sentence construction in some of the literary extracts is too tough, or making it the material for a dramatic team-teaching session, followed by small group work. Serious difficulty may well be experienced with immigrant groups, although one would have imagined that the motivation for such work might well stimulate the acquisition of improved language skills as well as to lessen the puzzlement due to the impact of new cultural mores and folkways (see also pages 88–9).

In his introduction to 'Relations between the Sexes', Stenhouse states that 'an understanding of the social and moral aspects of relations between the sexes cannot be achieved without a knowledge of the biology of sexuality and of the existence of techniques of birth control. This collection does not cover that ground . . .' This is where the Nuffield Secondary Science Project can fill a gap.

The Nuffield Secondary Science Project (13–16)

This project, for all ranges of ability from those just above remedial level to pupils capable of CSE Grade 1, is designed to encourage critical thinking and self-responsibility using wide experience of significant and relevant facts and concepts of science as the vehicle. It has produced resource materials for teachers on the exact sciences and some of the behavioural sciences too. The work is organized into eight themes and it is intended that teachers should choose work from all these to provide a balanced science course for the 13- to 16-year-old, through experience, discovery and investigation.

The themes germane to sex education are *Theme 3—The Biology of Man*, and *Theme 2—Continuity of Life*. Theme 2 deals with human heredity, world population and food problems, while in Theme 3 the whole of the human life cycle is considered, applying the principles of moral education laid down by Wilson not only to sex and adolescents but to old age and grandparents. Also in Theme 3 work is outlined on human behaviour, including the importance of the sex drives, and the criteria of moral education applied to international problems of overpopulation and pollution. Feasibility trials of part of Theme 3 were held in 15 schools for half a term. The first trial of the whole material was spread over 53 schools for one year—the material was then re-written taking cognisance of the feedback from the teachers. This second version was tried out for a year in 200 schools, suffered a second re-write and was finally published in May 1971, supported by school-tested and requested loop films and slides.

Work on marriage is not included as it was felt that this did indeed stray rather too far from the terms of reference of a science project. The physical basis of behaviour is dealt with at such crucial times of the life cycle as the effect of early or late development on adolescent behaviour, the effect of fluctuating hormone levels on adolescent girls and menopausal women, the physical changes which accompany ageing; pupils are encouraged to undertake voluntary work with the elderly, and greater realization of their handicaps increases understanding and promotes a more considerate way of life possibly for the pupils' grandparents too. Learning by experience of child development is recommended by the introduction of girls into playgroups and boys into infant classes in schools. Work is attempted on the different attitudes of boys and girls, unconscious use of trigger stimuli to copulatory behaviour and an examination of the unnecessary strength of the sex drive towards mating in modern society. 'Nevertheless, the mass media cash in on (a) its strength, (b) its lack of outlets and (c) its need for displacement stimuli.' This statement by Dennis Fox of Nottingham College of Education, the author of most of Theme 3, indicates the need for work on basic human drives which he has included. Pupils have identified drives appealed to by advertisements and have been incensed by their awareness of being 'got at'.

Thus not only are the basic anatomy and physiology dealt with (including a set of slides of human embryology), but they are related to behavioural aspects, and this is further extended into a simple study of human behaviour itself. Not unexpectedly, some science teachers feel unsuited to such work and an interdisciplinary approach is recommended. Again, teachers need to select from this material as they do in the Humanities Project; thus they are free to choose work on VD and contraception if they so desire, or conversely not include any of the work on the human life cycle at all.

Theme 3 does not provide a text book on the teaching of sex, but rather an outline of concepts and facts which are thought to be desirable and an indication of some methods by which they might be taught. An extensive list of references enables teachers to inquire further into aspects unfamiliar to them. Although background books for pupils are being produced, none of them deals with sex matters (see also p. 100).

The Schools Council Moral Education Curriculum Project

This project is based on the research of Peter McPhail on adolescence as a time of social experiment when they 'need to abandon a dependent relationship for an adult relationship with adults on terms of equality' (McPhail, 1967). This new relationship is sought by trying a variety of attitudes and actions which will produce reactions in individuals or groups. He found that 70 per cent of secondary school children expected the school to help them with their problems of relationships with individuals and with groups. 'Furthermore, boys and girls recognized the rewardingness of the considerate style of life in which consideration receives consideration in return' (McPhail, 1971).

Marylin Williams, working at Oxford in 1969, 'demonstrated a good, positive correlation between taking the role of the other and improving one's ability to treat the other person with consideration'. This is the basis of the project's material *In Other Peoples' Shoes* (*Lifeline*, 1972), which involves all the criteria for the moral education postulated by Wilson of the Farmington Trust. While McPhail acknowledges Wilson's work as an analytical tool, he considers that in the moral education of adolescents it is unrealistic to divide the work into separate skills to be developed in isolation from each other.

McPhail found that socially experimental learning reached a peak for girls at about 14 and for boys about a year later. With the raising of the school-leaving age to 16, the moral responsibility of the school to help adolescents understand what makes an action good or bad, and to help them do what is 'right', would become inescapable. He further states that 'we believe that moral education which does not help young people to greater health and happiness is at best no use, and that education in relationships which ignores sexual relationships is totally inadequate'. In fact, the work of this project has moved sex education from vague, woolly and widespread mumblings about personal relationships and morals by amateurs into the professional world of hypotheses supported by evidence, objectives stated in clear terms and their achievement by a variety of methods and pace, critically evaluated.

All the methods used involved imagination-role playing, writing poems and plays, expression through art-work, etc., making strip cartoons, collages, etc., as well as discussion of a variety of actions for any situation, and their possible consequences. Much of this is what the middle class child may get from its parents and one of the most important aspects of this project is that it succeeds in providing education for those most in need of moral education, i.e. those pupils who are conditioned to believe that anything goes as long as you don't get caught, that work is something to be skived, that property is something to be knocked off and that bashing the under-dog is the only thing that makes life tolerable. The project provides learning by experience in some very abstract concepts—the only way in which those of average intelligence and below are likely to learn such things. It makes a pleasant change in English education to see the non-academic child being catered for, as well as the top 20 per cent.

In Other Peoples' Shoes

This part of the project's work involves adolescents considering situations from their own point of view and from that of the one other person involved, and it would seem sensible to use this section before attempting the Humanities work on 'Relations between the Sexes', and also to precede both by the Nuffield Secondary Science Projects' work on the physical basis of behaviour. Heaven help the committed teacher who has to integrate all three—there will be many requests for sabbatical years just to read the material!

Fifteen examples are given of situations mostly concerned with male–female relationships and roles. The final section asks the individual to think about his or her own rights in a situation and is especially designed for those who are already considerate and self-negating. This is just as much of a problem in many adolescents as lack of consideration is in the majority. The following is one of the fifteen examples:

Situation 9. Sex roles: Boy friend/girl friend. You have a girl friend of whom you are extremely fond and she seems to care a lot about you. You suggest that you go off for a long day picnicing and walking in the school holidays. She seems reluctant to agree and you can't think why, as you know she enjoys walking.

What might (a) the boy's and (b) the girl's expectations be in this situation?

Should they discuss together how they see their relationship?

One can picture a lively session with boys taking the role of the girls and being corrected in no uncertain fashion. One of the 'Points of departure' loop films features a similar situation and it would be interesting to compare the effects of the two different techniques, while nevertheless remembering that neither gives a definite answer, but McPhail tops it by pointing out that in all these situations people may have to agree to differ; this is often a startling new concept to adolescents in the conformist stage.

Sensitivity Material

It is impossible to do justice to this soundly constructed and sophisticated work in such a short space, but briefly it is concerned with a problem situation and the individual has to decide what to do about it; it is imaginative social experiment for the class and an indication to the teacher of the level of maturity and the type of behaviour patterns to be found in the group. Furthermore, it neatly presents an outline of critical incidents contributing to the generation gap as well as boy/girl relationships and conflict with teachers. Situation 20, 'A teacher cannot keep order—what would you do?' should be used as sensitivity education for all student teachers; so should the appendix—a short course on recognizing non-verbal cues to other peoples' feelings.

Consequences

Here the consideration of the effects of a course of action or an attitude not just on an individual but on all others who might be affected by it. Parental care figures here and the following situations are suggested.

Outline what could happen if someone:

30. Leaves a child of four alone in a house.
33. Locks a child in a room.
43. Expects a child of five to find his own way home.

Again the centrality of this work suggests links with the Secondary Science work on learning about child care by experience in play-groups and the Humanities resource material on 'The Family'. This work also involves legal aspects which are all too often entirely omitted from sex education courses. The project is producing as part of its programme a book *I Didn't Know* on legal matters which pupils can use to predict some of the consequences of their actions.

The 78 situations suggested are not meant to be slogged through from start to finish. As in the Secondary Science Project, significance and relevance are the criteria for selection and teachers will always be able to think of better ideas of their own when presented with a set by other people. Also it is the habit of thought of considering consequences which is the objective here rather than a detailed knowledge of a variety of troublesome situations.

'Matinees and adult treatment in the classroom within a particular class goes oddly with school uniform, corporal punishment and dinner ladies employed to snoop around the girls' lavatories in search of smokers' wrote Anne Corbett in New Society (1970) of the Humanities Project; the same could be said of the Schools Council Moral Education Project.

The Schools Council General Studies Project

Liberal studies departments have one of the worst jobs in further education—their clientele is often typified by a lack of abstract thought, poor verbalization and can often only see the pragmatic aims of their education as relevant to their situation. With such a challenging situation it is perhaps not surprising that it is here that some of the best work in sex education has taken place. The motivation for the topic is high and a wide variety of educational objectives (from literacy, numeracy, including the interpretation of statistics and work on probability, verbal skills, using critical analysis of evidence in debate, and self-responsibility for pro-grammed work to emotional education) can be achieved by using the excellent work of the Schools Council General Studies Project (to be published in 1972). This project provides school-tested resources of some depth for liberal studies in sixth forms and colleges of further education.

The units are inter-related so that the selection given below is by no means exhaustive. There is a piece of semi-programmed learning on the contraceptive pill and sex hormones, including a consideration of the risks involved, using evidence from the Scowne report from a general survey on side effects of the Pill and from the IPPF. This last compares the death rate expected in a million women from pregnancy (2,600, plus 125 from legal abortions and 2,500 from criminal abortion) as opposed to death rates expected per million women on the Pill (23). There is also a unit on the future of birth control, including information about research in pills for men, prostaglandins (currently being investigated as early abortifacients) and alternatives to contraception as a means of population control such as homosexuality and financial disincentives. Add to this the unit on world population, the work book on world population, units on world population and food, and economic underdevelopment and it will be readily understood that superficiality is the last sin of which this project can be accused. In fact it may be accused of committing the frequent British educational sin of academic snobbism, being more suited in language, habits of thought and perseverance needed to the academic sixth rather than to the technical apprentice or the day release shop assistant. For these the Humanities Project would seem to provide shorter pieces of more compulsive reading. But this is carping criticism and does not take into account the excellence of the teacher; liberal studies teachers *have* to be excellent to survive.

This material has been produced by experienced teachers and school-tested—but even the most inexperienced could not fail to get a class going on the right lines on the unit entitled 'Sex education, whether and if so, how?' which ranges from the Schofield report (a succinct summary), the Newsom report, A. S. Neill, one of our anti-sex education psychiatrists, and a Victorian doctor, to a simulation exercise of a school staff discussion on how to introduce sex education. Units on abortion, and genetic engineering are also included, but perhaps the most outstanding is that on 'Making love', a selection of love poems of great sensitivity and insight (see also p. 68).

51

Like the Humanities Project and the Nuffield Secondary Science Project, the General Studies Project does not support the naive philosophy of 'Give them the facts and let them make up their minds'; it provides the skills and teaching method necessary before the making up of minds is possible, however many facts are known.

Youth work

The Albemarle Report gave a great impetus to the emergence of youth clubs based on social counselling rather than on ping pong and athletic activities. These clubs provide a place for young people to meet and talk apart from street corners, doorways, commercial coffee bars and pubs. A typical club would provide a constant canteen including facilities for members to cook (and wash up) their own meals for the cost of the materials, and perhaps a place to change from work clothes to going-out gear, a place for girls to experiment with make-up and hair styles. Some even provided a graffiti wall, which was painted over when too full or too obscene, but which concentrated all such efforts into one place—a device now used on Swedish housing complexes. The essential provision, however, was for a variety of communicating adults to be on tap for discussions about everything from comparative religion to sex.

The sex education provided was informal and individual; group activities such as the showing of films or special discussion sessions grew out of informal requests and were in no sense courses laid on. At the 1948 raising of the school-leaving age from 14–15, those adolescents who were unwillingly forced to stay on in school and caused much trouble in the formal teaching situations there were often found to be the most interested in suggesting group activity ideas in the informal club situation. One such club was the Healey Teen Bar in Sheffield under the direction of Edrie Green. Here the basic counselling work not only helped to produce a considerate way of life in sexual matters but also led, for example, to youths going to the Peak District on Saturdays to build up the walls of sheep runs which they might previously have thoughtlessly broken down. Such clubs may look too disorganized and untidy for those who hold the purse strings and who have forgotten how much pressure is needed to induce one teenager to tidy his bedroom, let alone a club used by hundreds of them each of whom can put the blame for untidiness on someone else. They have been said to encourage the 'wrong type'. One leader was told that she should be doing something 'for the better girls' rather than wasting her time with the rowdies. The social and personal education which such clubs provide cannot be easily assessed. 'Just talking' seems a waste of the ratepayers' money to many unaware of the real value of such places for letting off emotional as well as physical steam. Many have been closed down because of complaints about noise from neighbours and because lack of understanding of the complex and highly professional job which they try to do. Nevertheless, those which manage to survive do an excellent job in providing the extra parental counsellor which adolescents need (see page 96) and were early pioneers in informed, individual sex education.

The chief advantage of such 'street corners with a roof on' clubs is that they attract the early maturers often from apathetic homes and thus have the opportunity of giving sex education to those who need it most in counselling situations. Many youth organizations are acutely aware of their responsibilities in this field and have been running courses of some depth for the training of youth leaders in sex education for some time, long before the education committees (with a few notable exceptions) began to form working parties on the subject.

References

ALBERMARLE REPORT (1960). *The Youth Service in England and Wales.* CMND 929. London: HMSO.

ANDREY, A. C. and SCHEPPS, S. (1969). *How Babies Are Made.* Netherlands: Time/Life.

ASHLEY MONTAGU, C. (1968). *Man and Aggression.* Oxford: OUP.

BRITISH BROADCASTING CORPORATION (1971). *School Broadcasting and Sex Education in the Primary School*, from 35, Marylebone High Street, London, W1M 4AA. 18p.

CHANTER, A. (1966). *Sex Education in the Primary School.* London: Macmillan.

EXETER EDUCATION COMMITTEE (1970). *Scheme of Education in Personal Relationships*, from City Education Office, 33, St. David's Hill, Exeter, EX4 4DE. 5p.

GRAMPIAN TELEVISION (1968). 'Living and Growing.' *A Report on a Sex Education Series for Primary Schools*, from Queen's Cross, Aberdeen, AB9 2XJ.

GRAMPIAN TELEVISION (1970). *A Report on the Repeat Transmission of 'Living and Growing' in the Grampian Region, Spring Term, 1970.* Duplicated copy, SAC/3/(71).

McPHAIL, P. (1967). Notes for a paper to the British Psychological Society, London Conference.

McPHAIL, P. (1971). Letter to the Health Education Journal.

NEURATH, M. (1965). Various illustrated books for primary schools, e.g. *How Life Begins.* London: Max Parrish.

NUFFIELD 'O' LEVEL BIOLOGY (1966). *Teachers' Guide I: Introducing Living Things.* London: Longmans/Penguin.

NUFFIELD SECONDARY SCIENCE (1971). *Theme 2—The Continuity of Life. Theme 3—The Biology of Man.* London: Longmans.

REID, D. and BOOTH, P. (1970). *How Life Begins.* London: Heinemann.

SCHOOLS COUNCIL GENERAL STUDIES PROJECT. (To be published in 1972.) Inquiries should be made to the Secretary, General Studies Project, The King's Manor, York.

SCHOOLS COUNCIL MORAL EDUCATION CURRICULUM PROJECT: LIFELINE (1972). McPhail, P.: *In Other Peoples' Shoes.*
Chapman, H.: *Proving the Rule?*
Ungoed-Thomas, J.: *What Would You Have Done?*
Ungoed-Thomas, J.: *Our School.*
McPhail, P., Chapman, H. and Ungoed-Thomas, J.: *Our School.* London: Longmans.

Films

BRITISH BROADCASTING CORPORATION: Merry-go-round programmes; from BBC TV Enterprises, Villiers House, Haven Green, London, W5. And for hire from BBC TV Enterprises, Film Hire, 25, The Burroughs, Hendon, London, NW4.

EOTHEN, 'Points of Departure' Loop Films. Available from Sound Services, 209 Kingston Road, London S.W.19.

Teaching Aids

SCHOOLS COUNCIL HUMANITIES PROJECT (1970). 'Relations Between the Sexes.' 'The Family.' Teachers' kits. London: Heinemann. £10 each.

CHAPTER THREE

Other Agencies Concerned with Sex Education

A VERY FULL but concise treatment of the variety of agencies at work in this field, including a succinct summary of all Governmental reports and of the work of many LEA's, is given in the proceedings of a working group of the International Planned Parenthood Federation held in Tunis in 1969 entitled *Responsible Parenthood and Sex Education* (Burke, 1969). This section therefore merely adds to what has already been said in this book and brings it up-to-date as much as possible. Incidentally, the book also provides an outline of international sex education programmes and their evaluation; it is comforting to note that the best of English sex education is far in advance of the general international scene, which is still concerned mainly with the anatomy and physiology of sex, and wandering in a confusion of thought about relationships and morals.

One of the problems of sex education in school is that the teacher cannot be expected to be an expert on every aspect of the human life cycle. In a very adequate lesson dealing with birth, a young male teacher confessed he felt that some of his answers to the class's questions were very thin and that he would welcome more information on the subject. Opinion is gradually turning to the point of view that teachers should be able to fill such informational gaps individually through the use of resources centres, not merely equipped with books and films, but with programmed work for self-instruction, used in conjunction with individual tutorials. Eventually this and perhaps also the specialist help offered by a number of national agencies may replace the traditional courses, where relatively formal methods are used. The teacher needs to consult the specialist to ensure that simplification does not mean superficiality, and hence that early concepts do not have to be unlearned when it is possible for the learner to deal with more complex ideas. Many agencies provide 'trained' lecturers for schools and colleges; but relatively few of them know very much about the provision of active learning situations, and while many are excellent, the quality varies enormously.

The National Childbirth Trust

Often erroneously called the 'Natural' Childbirth Trust, this organization trains its own teachers especially to help women negate the Biblical idea that children are born in sorrow and pain. Perhaps the best evaluation of their work is by the number of mothers who once having been taught how to work with their bodies instead of against them, have become NCT teachers themselves. The Trust also gives training in behavioural aspects as well as anatomical and physiological methods. Its critics say that the hypotheses underlying the Trust's work is purely pragmatic and unsupported by evidence. It is nevertheless irrefutable that their methods reduce the sum total of human misery and it is interesting to speculate that the criticism may stem from problems of authority and control, i.e. removing these attributes from the doctor and the midwife and giving them to the mother.

The Trust's work, though biased towards birth also extends into the field of general sex education, and they have run film sessions for adolescents and produce a catalogue of resource material. Perhaps their most useful function is in bringing people together in their study days for teachers. These are informal discussions and lectures in some depth on a small group basis, where teachers can exchange ideas with film makers, local authority health education workers, advisers and inspectors and university and college lecturers. Contacts made through NCT study days have improved the circulation of knowledge and methods (there is a great need for centralization here) and incidentally improved the standard of many sex education training courses in schools, colleges and universities. The Trust has contributed much to the integration and co-ordination of the experience of workers in a wide variety of fields in sex education and has shown itself willing to learn from others.

The Family Planning Association

Like the NCT, the FPA is biased towards one aspect of sex education, but it has always been interested in the field as a whole and has appointed an education officer (1971) for the promotion of wider activities. Apart from its work in the provision of clinics and training its staff, it provides trained lecturers for schools and colleges and is renowned for the excellent and comprehensive book shop in Mortimer Street, London W.1, which also runs a first-class postal service and keeps an up-to-date list of stock available.

From the FPA's many projects two are particularly worthy of note: The Community Education Project for South London, under the chairmanship of Dr. John McEwan, with David Barnard as the Educational Organizer, and Dr. Tunnadine's use of the psycho-physical therapy methods of Dr. Michael Balint in a very individual exercise in sex education in the field of female sexual anxiety.

Dr. Tunnadine and her colleagues examined their own techniques as family planning doctors and also their own prejudices as well as the problems of 20,000 patients and began to explore the little known fundamentals behind all requests for contraceptive help, trying to understand the patient's communication in depth. 'The unwarned and unheralded onset of menstruation . . . particularly when the only information has come not from the mother, but from the salacious reports of giggling school-fellows' is reported as one of the causes of emotional upset by Dr. Tunnadine in her book *Contraception and Sexual Life* (1970). Furthermore, she states that 'we find that without the exploration of fantasy and anxiety . . . factual teaching, however warmly and encouragingly done, can only be accepted and taken by individual patients according to their own emotional capacity. This may be of interest to those who must decide how and when to instruct their young. The fear is that too much knowledge too soon encourages them to go forth and experiment. To illustrate that for many this is not so, we cite a group of patients who were all professional women with ample factual knowledge who nevertheless were emotionally unable to use their knowledge.' A comforting piece of evidence for the sex educator.

The Family Planning Association's Community Education Project for South London (*Educational Organizer, David Barnard*)

This was an ambitious project to educate all levels of the community in family planning, including contraception. Factual knowledge of contraception cannot stand alone. It must be supported often by attitude change and some knowledge of its psychosexual aspects as well as an examination of the practical problems of supply and availability. It is only realistic to aver that the project passed on a good deal of information on these aspects, stimulated discussion where the ground was potentially favourable, but changed few attitudes at the decision-making level of the community.

There seems to be among certain age and culture groups of 'decision makers' an attitude which considers that ignorance is the best defence against pre-marital sex, and this includes ignorance of contraceptives. Whatever the reason, relatively few local authorities have implemented the National Health Service (Family Planning) Act 1967 which empowered them to establish their own family planning clinics. Lawrence Green in his prize-winning essay, 'Identifying and overcoming barriers to the diffusion of knowledge about family planning', says, 'At the community level, decisions affecting public access to family planning information and services are legislated or administered according to the spread of knowledge beyond the scientific and professional levels. Knowledge at this level . . . is a major determinant of access to knowledge at the ultimate levels of couples and individuals.' Thus Green's experience in East Pakistan parallels David Barnard's in South London.

Although many of the meetings inspired by this project were to result in little or no official implementation of the working group's conclusions for education in schools, others resulted in action, both by individuals and by groups. Thus the project provided, or added to, the necessary impetus for training sessions to be held for teachers and for serious discussion on facts and methods not only in contraception education but in sex education as a whole.

Incidentally, when project speakers visited schools by invitation, both the naivety and the sophistication of the questions they were asked were surprising; the range was from 'Can you use Tampax if you have an IUD?' to 'Does the Pill damage the pituitary gland?' In the project's work in colleges of education, 14 talks were given, nine being requested by students and five requested by staff. While this is undoubtedly due to the fact that many colleges take their responsibilities in this field seriously, it appears that the students were more enthusiastic than the staff.

Perhaps the best educational idea to emerge from the project, although it was never implemented, was the draft scheme of unit courses in all aspects of sex education. This is fully outlined in the final report of the project, McEwan and Barnard, *Towards an Educational Policy in Family Planning* (1970). Accepting that sex education is necessarily interdisciplinary, and that all teachers are not expected to teach such parts of the course with which they feel personal difficulties, the project suggested a series of units, which could be selected by individuals to suit their own needs—biologists might opt for units on morals and cultural differences, while divinity specialists might prefer those dealing with facts.

Apart from a tendency to think of passive methods of education rather than involving the recipients in decision-making processes, this project produced a large amount of excellent work on a very small budget and it is sad to realize that so many of the activities it began (e.g. the up-dating courses for health visitors, midwives and nurses, the introductory courses for social workers) were left in mid-air at the end of the two years of its life.

Brook Advisory Centres

These centres not only give contraceptive advice to the young and unmarried but do so with the stated aims of inculcating a sense of sexual responsibility and of mitigating the suffering caused by unwanted pregnancy and illegal abortion. Their work is therefore remedial, picking up the pieces left by the lack of sex education amongst those who most need it.

The centres have come under heavy criticism which accuses them of encouraging pre-marital sex. It is apparent that while they do encourage the responsible and considerate way of life, side effects must occur and it is difficult to evaluate the sum total of 'good' done, if only because the definition of 'good' in this case is unlikely to be agreed by the protagonists. In one college of education in the north-west it was reported that since a Brook Centre opened in its vicinity, it was the done thing to be seen queuing there, wearing a college scarf, as a sign of sexual maturity. Again, the centre can only have been one factor in the social pressures within the college to conform to a putative sexual norm.

The centres are truly advisory and not merely contraceptive

supermarkets, but it seems a pity that such sex education, which must of necessity often be too little and too late, is needed at all, nor perhaps will it be when the rest of the agencies concerned both in school and society are doing a fully professional job in the field.

The International Planned Parenthood Federation

Both the international headquarters of this organization and its European office are situated in London and both provide facilities for investigation of data concerned with demography and all aspects of family planning, including sex education, from almost all the countries in the world. For example, the headquarters library at 18 Lower Regent Street, London, has a large and comprehensive selection of American and British textbooks and journals on sex education, as well as a film, filmstrip, model, poster and slide reference library.

IPPF also produce a newsletter and several publications which have included for example an excellent map of the pituitary region annotated with research references reporting the evidence for the functions of the various parts, including their effects on sexual mechanisms. Work in science and an academic course in human ecology are included in the soft-covered book *Population education and the younger generation* (Lawton, 1971), which is a report of a course held by IPPF in London for those involved in such work from Pakistan, India, Ceylon and Afghanistan.

Local education authorities

Space does not permit a survey of the many working parties' reports, syllabuses for all ages of children, the provision of resources centres, the organization of specialist help from doctors, health visitors, etc., and selection and training methods for teachers undertaken by LEA's. ILEA is the first authority to produce its own television programmes on sex education: 'Lifeline' for 11-year-olds and 'Threshold' for the colleges of further education and sixth forms (details of programmes from ILEA ETV, Tennyson Street, London S.W.8); and it has recently appointed two curriculum developers in the field of child care.

The Gloucestershire Association for Family Life is, however, unique; it was formed in 1962 and consists not only of the officials from the LEA but also individuals and representatives of a wide variety of organizations concerned with 'secure and happy family life as a basis of a stable and civilized community' and 'a greater understanding of the behaviour and beliefs of other people'. The group includes representatives from both Catholic and Protestant religions, social workers, youth organizations, WEA, WI and TWG, from medicine and from the Magistrates' Association, as well as from the police and the colleges of education, the local education authorities and local health authorities both for the city and the county. This is in fact an educational project underwritten by all sections of the community—and remarkably, one which has been running successfully for ten years. This education in personal relationships is for all sections of the community, not only in schools but in youth work, women's groups, student counselling, parent–teacher groups and industrial training schemes. The Association recruits and trains people for the work, disseminates information and publicizes its aims and activities, thus ensuring extension of its work as well as financial support and public approval.

The work of the Association links and overlaps with the extensive scheme of education in personal relationships in secondary schools. From the beginning, the Association and the county authority has set sex education in the wider context of the considerate way of life and all aspects of growing up, from the difficulties encountered when first going to work to the problems involved in living with Gran. A brief account of the work in Gloucestershire is available (The Gloucestershire Scheme for Education in Personal Relationships and Family Life, The Third Report and Handbook, 1971).

One can quibble with minor points in the scheme. For example, with earlier maturity, 11 may be too late to prepare some children for the changes of puberty. Nevertheless it is remarkable, not only for the soundness of its basic concepts but also for the persistance with which it has been refined and extended over the years with a degree of astringent self-criticism which is rare in educational circles.

The Association has undertaken attitude surveys (1966) among young people, but no formal investigation into the effects of their work. Perhaps the best evaluation is that the work grows and continues, unhampered by sensationalism. An interesting sociological research project lies in Gloucestershire for those interested in the change effected in the public debate on sex education by the Association's work; comparison of attitudes expressed in newspapers in this and other countries could prove interesting.

Local health authorities

Many of these provide a health education department which includes sex education among its other activities. In the best of these departments a resources centre exists, with supplies of posters, pamphlets and models; often a graphics technician is employed to produce materials requested by the visiting health teachers. These go into schools, colleges, factories, when asked, and also run their own classes for young parents, teachers and the general public. In some areas they have taken on the task of introducing sex education to parents in the school situation.

A criticism usually levelled at local authority health educators dealing with sex education is that they lecture, without a full knowledge of the individual variation within the classes and without due regard for levels of communication. This may well apply to some but the majority are well aware of their use as counsellors from outside the school environment, which many school children welcome.

Lack of co-ordination within the schools visited is also a problem —the health educator may be faced with adolescents who have already heard what she is going to say. On the other hand, teachers often complain that they are not allowed to know what the health educator has done; presumably the intention here is to safeguard the confidentiality of the questions she has had to deal with, but it would seem that more discussion between the school and its visitors would bring benefits all round.

It is perhaps invidious to name particular centres of excellence in LHA's but from the work of the Croydon Department has come a useful book *Health Education—Patterns for Teaching* (Elliott and May, 1969) which is particularly good on child development, and from Sheffield a well-organized piece of work on the venereal diseases (see page 82). The role of the LHA's therefore is not merely of providing sex education specialists for those who are without them, but also in innovation in the field of communication methods and the provision of support, resources and training for teachers.

Research into why they are asked to give help and also into negative reactions to this help might well be rewarding.

National television: its contribution to the public debate

One of the first programmes made by the BBC on the birth of a baby did not actually show the birth itself except in still photographs (1958), but in 1960 a filmed birth was shown with a preliminary announcement for susceptible viewers; a large number of protesting letters were received.

However, in 1968 (repeated in 1969) another programme on birth attracted only one letter of protest and that anonymous; the BBC has taken a gradualist approach and moved with the changing climate of public opinion, nevertheless being sometimes slightly ahead of it in the eyes of certain viewers. The 1968 programme drew letters of appreciation—in particular requests that such programmes be shown for husbands as well as wives. This indicates a great change in attitudes from the earlier programmes which drew protests about the invasion of feminine privacy.

The part played by national television in providing both material and authority for reasoned discussion on sexual matters in its excellent programmes on VD, contraception and world population and recently male and female roles in a number of cultures, as well as on birth and child development, has perhaps been the most significant and effective factor in adult and parent education.

The same cannot be said about the level of discussion which any of the national television presenters have produced about sex education itself, most of which have been superficial in the extreme. Many have degenerated into slanging matches between sharply polarized opinions, leaving anger in the hearts of participants and viewers alike and contributing little except stimulation to the public debate. While one sees the need for the representation of all shades of opinion, television presenters are rarely schooled in the techniques of managing a high level of critical discussion with what amounts to a non-streamed class. While television budgets half-a-million pounds for series of programmes on history, culture and who-dunnits, sex education gets the superficial journalistic treatment which the various companies feel it deserves. Desmond Wilcox, Editor of 'Man Alive', which held a discussion on 'Sex and Common

63

Sense' in June 1971, replying to listeners' letters in the *Radio Times*, said 'It's my own—older—generation—which seems to get noisy, didactic and abusive about sex'; it is to be hoped that television will eventually refuse to offer its considerable authority to the presentation of such views which appear to be based on little else but emotion.

It might be more instructive to separate the protagonists—to produce an anti-sex educationist programme and one devoted totally to the pro-sex education group—at least viewers could then make an unimpeded assessment of the degrees of psychological freedom present. It would also be pleasant if the costly gatherings of experts in the field were more efficiently used—each one seems to get a few minutes of *ad hoc* commentary and no time to state underlying philosophies in any depth. It would also be useful to have an instructional programme on the myths and fallacies accompanying much of the naive debate, for example that ignorance is more likely to lead to sexual experiment than full knowledge. It is not surprising that many people in the sex education field refuse invitations to appear on such programmes, either on TV or local radio. Many who do, never accept another.

Although the overall picture is depressing, at least ITV's 'What Shall we Tell the Children' made a useful and valid attempt to explore why parents did not educate their families in sexual matters and Grampian TV produced a series 'Talk About Sex' for parents in 1970. The four programmes began with pre-adolescent education and the difficulties of parents who have never found it easy to communicate with their children on such matters, even although they knew the appropriate facts and vocabulary. Ludovic Kennedy discussed this matter with Dr. Dennis (who presented the 'Living and Growing' programmes), who himself admitted to the Eugenics Society in 1970 that he found difficulty in talking to his own family about homosexuality. In the second programme a young mother discussed her problems, while in the third adults listen to a group of young people talking about such explosive questions as how late they should stay out and how far they should go. The final programme was aimed at helping parents to assess their own standards and beliefs against those of today's young generation.

The programmes have not been evaluated and it is unlikely that they will be seen in England.

The press: women's magazines and newspapers

National and local newspapers ensure that children need to know about sex; in addition they play a varied part in the public debate from the plain ludicrous to the highly informative and critical. The *Daily Mirror* is perhaps unique in that it gave double-page coverage to the Health Education Council's leaflet setting out the various means of contraceptives, their failure rates and risks.

One of the main sources of evaluation of sex education is the thousands of letters which pour in each week not only to the *Daily Mirror* but to various magazines for women and girls. To conclude that so many women and girls prefer to ask a stranger for advice on sexual matters is not entirely true—the columnists show themselves to be far more understanding and confidential than friends and neighbours might be. They are also people to whom (like Family Planning Clinic doctors) one is *allowed* to talk about sex. It is interesting to speculate that these letters may be only the tip of the iceberg; it takes resolution, literacy and high motivation to write a letter, *not* tear it up and then actually post it. At a conservative estimate (some magazines are unwilling to divulge this information) the various advice columns in women's magazines dealing with sexual problems receive an average of 1,000 letters per week. Between them, this makes a staggering total of at least 60,000 per year, indicating a vast need for knowledge and a situation about which no sex educator can afford to be complacent. Such outlets were not generally available to men until the Marjorie Proops Column began in the *Daily Mirror* in 1971; in its first six months the column received between 700–800 letters per week, of which about 25 per cent were from men.

In their articles on sex, child development and marriage, women's magazines do an excellent job. The articles are written in simple but carefully researched language (in strong contrast to many health education pamphlets on similar subjects), are well laid out and illustrated and do not shirk the more difficult problems of pre-marital intercourse as they once did. Magazines for young girls discuss behavioural problems using stories and strip cartoons which on the whole give a very realistic approach to problems girls are likely to meet.

Such realism is less apparent in the stories in women's magazines,

C

however, which take a decidedly rosy outlook on sex, marriage and babies. Fantasy is what the public wants and so they get it; why should the weary housewife be denied her favourite opiate? Unfortunately, these magazines are also read by young girls who take this fantasy world for reality, and when the ugly duckling meets her handsome prince (who realizes her true worth although she is not so glamorous as she might be) in the real world she may well be left with an unwanted pregnancy. The effect of romantic stories and novels on the formation of norms of behaviour by those who have no other source of information is unestimated, but evidence seems to point to many who have had to learn the difference between fact and fiction in a very hard way. There are some, particularly social workers, who consider that romantic fiction 'depraves' more than does pornography.

There is much scope for investigation in the effect of magazines on behaviour; it is believed that magazines may be bought for example for the sake of the reassurance they give that the casserole's in the oven (preferably in colour), and all's right with the world—and the comforting thought that there are always those worse off than you, mediated by the agony columns. James Hemming (*Problems of Adolescent Girls*, 1960) surveyed a small sample of girls' questions from a magazine which ran a letter column only sporadically in 1960 and found that one of the major problems was security of self-image. As Agnete Breastrup, President of IPPF, puts it, they seek the answer to two questions, 'Will I become a normal adult?', 'Will I be accepted as a partner by the opposite sex?' At least the women's magazines have reassured thousands of girls on a point of anatomy—it is quite normal to have a clitoris, although sex education textbooks rarely give evidence that anyone has one. However, today the clitoris is featuring in school textbooks.

References

BURKE, S. (ed.) (1969). *Responsible Parenthood and Sex Education*, from IPPF, 18, Lower Regent Street, London SW1. 75p.

ELLIOTT, D. and MAY, E. (1969). *Health Education—Patterns for Teaching*. London: Macmillan.

GLOUCESTERSHIRE ASSOCIATION FOR FAMILY LIFE (1966). *Survey on Attitudes to Religious, Health and Sex Education*. Loan copies available from GAFL, 2, College Street, Gloucester, GL1 2NE.

GLOUCESTERSHIRE ASSOCIATION FOR FAMILY LIFE (1971). *The Third Annual Report and Handbook*. Education Department, Shire Hall, Gloucester. 15p.

GREEN, L. (1970). 'Identifying and overcoming barriers to the diffusion of knowledge about family planning.' *Advances in Fertility Control*, **5,** 2 (reprinted in *J. Inst. Health Educ.*, **19,** 1).

HEMMING, J. (1960). *Problems of Adolescent Girls*. London: Heinemann. Out of print.

INNER LONDON EDUCATION AUTHORITY EDUCATIONAL TELEVISION SERVICE. *Lifeline*, from ILEA ETV Centre, Tennyson Street, London SW8.

LAWTON, D. (ed.) (1971). *Population Education and the Younger Generation*, from IPPF, 18, Lower Regent Street, London SW1. 95p.

MCEWAN, V. and BARNARD, D. (1970). *Towards an Educational Policy in Family Planning*, from FPA Community Education Project for South London, 160, Peckahm Rye, London SE22. 20p.

TUNNADINE, L. P. D. (1970). *Contraception and Sexual Life*. London: Tavistock.

Films

TELEVISION PROGRAMMES:
GRANADA (1969). 'What Shall We Tell the Children?'
GRAMPIAN (1970). 'Talking about Sex.'

CHAPTER FOUR

Particular Problems

Visual symbolism in sex education: the use of models and film

SEX EDUCATORS are often those who have had further education in Biology, if not some medical or paramedical training and are used to the visual symbolism of the anatomical textbook.

They become expert at adding a three-dimensional interpretation to a two-dimensional diagram, adding colours to help identify what would otherwise appear as sets of parallel tramlines; they also acquire the skill of interpreting numerical indications of scale and of being able to relate a diagram to its place in the human body.

Unfortunately many of the children receiving sex education do not possess these skills, and many have not perhaps reached the necessary level of mental development to enable these skills to develop. A large picture of a sperm revolted one class, as it looked more like a snake or a worm than anything which one would like to have in one's insides. After seeing a film loop, a description of menstruation given by one girl which was agreed with by most members of her class, 'Well, you see there's this ping pong ball which rolls down the tubes and rips out the lining of the uterus'. Others have had to be convinced that their Fallopian tubes were not purple and did not have white tacking stitches running down them. Relating the size of the uterus to reality and demonstrating its position in the body have also created difficulties, as the uterus in one much-used loop film looks as if it had been given wings (the fimbriated ends of the Fallopian tubes) and is about to take off in flight. While in the hands of the experienced teacher, who is aware of the lack of visually sophisticated interpretation in the class, such films can be useful, too many tyros are unaware of the difficulties which such diagrams pose. The IPPF in its attempts to educate populations with a low general level of education is possibly more aware of these problems than most and has a collection of excellent, transportable, three-dimensional models for teaching anatomical details. Many teachers also reinforce work from diagrams and films by encouraging pupils to make simple three-dimensional models of what they have seen, but in plasticene rather than using ping-pong balls and detergent bottles as recommended in a book for science teachers. The use of any model must always be accompanied by asking the class how it is *not* like the real thing, and this must be done with highly-coloured two-dimensional diagrams too.

Lack of feedback from young classes is often responsible for the continued recommendation of some poor films and film strips; teachers are simply not aware of the confusion left in the minds of the class. In contrast, when working with student teachers or in-service courses, feedback is usually uninhibited—when the film 'Half a Million Teenagers' is screened a roar of laughter usually greets the visual symbolism used to show the transmission of VD by sexual intercourse. Figures float across the screen and, as they come in contact, cross-hatching appears on the pelvic region. This euphemism leaves 14-year-olds in little doubt of what is meant, although the teacher must ensure that all appreciate it, and it does not disturb tetchy aldermen on education committees at all.

Omnibus sex films

There was a vogue for these in the late 1960's—50-minute films, or even longer, showing birth, intercourse, menstruation, anatomy and perhaps a touch of the emotional side, often represented by the couple walking by the seashore for no apparent reason. This is the visual equivalent of the short sharp talk mentioned earlier and just as educationally superficial. The latest in this genre is, of course, Martin Cole's 'Growing Up'; this film, like all the others, proceeds to dispense knowledge speedily and superficially like a visual lecture, expecting no feedback and only allowing a full discussion if it is shown in small sections. Today and particularly in sex education, 'teaching' is subordinated to learning; for example, today's teachers are educated to outline the objectives which their work should achieve and none of the omnibus films have seriously considered this. In Cole's film, the objectives behind the notorious masturbation sequences are obscure. Most children discover this activity for themselves at an early age. If they do not masturbate, it is likely that they have been inhibited from doing so by social pressures and it is doubtful whether the film would remove such inhibitions. Conversely, it is obviously also of little use to those already masturbating—therefore why include it? There is only one danger in masturbation and that is from infection by dirty fingers —yet in Cole's film a boy is shown touching his penis with grubby fingernails. Similarly, the dull, somewhat mechanistic, norm of intercourse established by the film provoke groans and cynical laughter in a students' union in Wales. Adolescents really do want to know what intercourse is like (see page 95), and if the desired objective is to inform about the nature of such a variable experience, the whole range should be covered from Desmond Morris's full description in *The Naked Ape* to the excellent source unit of the General Studies Project on 'Making love', a selection of poems which give brilliant insight, particularly those of E. E. Cummings and Ted Hughes. First-class film is obviously of use here, too, but all resources should be used with the *caveat* that it is impossible to communicate the whole picture, and that everyone will have his own individual experience which will itself vary enormously from time to time. To establish a norm is to deny the enjoyable variety possible within intercourse and to place crippling demands upon adolescents who have not reached their full sexual identity. Oddly enough, an omnibus film appears in the Humanities List, the Dutch film 'Sex is Everywhere', where sexual behaviour (even masturbation) is represented, somewhat cryptically for all except balleto-manes, by go-go dancers. The excellence of the film in the original Dutch is in the interviews given by adolescents about their sexual experience; one young man admits that when he and his girl got into bed they didn't quite know what to do, so they read *Winnie the Pooh*! Some good discussion about the urge to conform and to get to bed, even when you don't know what to do when you get there, might follow if it had not been forgotten after the tedious 50 minutes spent watching the film. It takes a Zefirelli to hold attention and story line for that length of time; health educators would do better to stick to ten-minute single concept films.

The emotional impact of films

Some years ago the sponsors of the film on the birth of a baby 'To Janet a Son?' used to send round a representative to see if those showing the film were capable of dealing with the emotions aroused and making it clear that the company accepted no responsibility in the matter. One such gentleman admitted that he himself had passed out during the showing of the animated diagram section on birth! But there are many people who are affected simply by the colour of blood and the peculiar unfamiliar blue of the cyanosed baby as it emerges from the mother. Most audiences exhibit tension with this film, cigarettes are rapidly smoked, enormous gales of laughter greet some of the midwifely pronouncements, and it is useful for the person showing the film in some audiences to switch off and relieve the tension with laughter where possible. The film has a long introduction on ante-natal care, and this, too, is useful where audiences are unused to the sight of the naked human body; the film introduces it gradually (too coyly for some) and works up gradually to the emotional climax. Several teachers switch off the sound track altogether and make their own commentary, largely because of the very middle class accents and terms of speech used.

Colour films produce more emotion than black and white, but this can be helpful where a disturbed member of the class can talk out with the teacher just why the film has had such an effect. Apart from this, little useful generalization can be made about the emotional effect of film. The Swedish film 'Barnet—The Child' was shown to a group of Biology teachers in training, two of whom found it emotionally upsetting, one felt it was the best material he'd seen for the prevention of irresponsible fatherhood, and all disliked the visual symbolism used to represent the muscles of the uterus (which looked rather like surgical stitching and were very misleading). The emotion was largely due to the fact that birth is shown from the midwife's point of view—unless a mother is using a mirror she sees very little except the baby's emergence. The biologists could see little point in using the film. They preferred to use Jane Madder's 'Birth, a Family Affair', which shows, in black and white, birth from the mother's point of view, with a relaxed father assisting her in a moment of cramp (as opposed to the Swedish film where the father looks as if he is totally unnecessary on the scene) and with the older children coming in to see the new baby. They felt 'To Janet a Son?' might be used to demonstrate the fact that hospitals are not necessarily hostile environments.

However, a very experienced teacher in further education much

71

prefers 'Barnet', and for a variety of very good reasons. Similarly, a group of teachers looking at the now out-of-date film 'Learning to Live' expressed the following views:

'The music is unsuitable.'

'The music is exactly right.'

'I would use this film as an introduction.'

'I would use this film as a drawing together at the end of the course.'

'This film is too advanced for 13- to 15-year-olds.'

'This film is suitable for secondary modern school pupils aged 14–16.'

All of this underlines the necessity for teachers to see films themselves first and to decide whether they fit the needs of their own particular class. Is the film consolidatory or introductory? One of the best omnibus films is McGraw Hill's 'Human Reproduction', but while it is too lengthy for an introduction it is too superficial for use in consolidation. On the other hand, the first part of 'To Janet a Son?' is an excellent revision and reinforcement of previously learned physiology, although rarely used as such. In teaching about contraception, motivation is a further objective for film selection, particularly in developing countries. Other films are made for use after motivation has been achieved, for example to familiarize women with clinic procedures and facilitate social skills enabling them to get contraceptive advice without personal embarrassment or fear of social censure.

Too often in sex education, film has been used to give a cloak of darkness to an embarrassed teacher and to do a perfunctory job to a whole class rather than to aid learning in a group of individuals, communicating with another well-informed individual.

Finally, one of the dangers of birth films is that they establish an unattainable norm; not every woman is capable of enjoying childbirth. While it is essential that birth sequences do show the overwhelming and ecstatic feelings of the mother when she sees her child for the first time, it is important that girls should not feel that they have to enjoy every minute of labour.

Emotional identification with film

When one girl in a group has had an illegitimate pregnancy, or found that intercourse is unsatisfactory or has been infected with VD and shared her experiences with others in the group, it might seem that they would learn from her troubles. On the contrary, the group, while publicly showing charity and concern, in private rarely identify with the victim, seeing her as stupid, unlucky, or ignorant and are quite certain that such things will not happen to them.

When, however, they can see a film and identify with a character in it, vicariously sharing his or her emotions, this can educate with enormous impact, and adolescents can feel intensely what it is like to have to tell your boy friend that you are pregnant, to be left to support your children, to try to be both father and mother to a child. Even where the way of life depicted is far different from that experienced by the class, with a sensitive teacher much can be achieved, although the nearer the culture and accents of the film actors are to those of the class the easier is the identification. Showing the National Film Board of Canada's 'Phoebe' in a school with 50 per cent Indian immigrants resulted in great understanding, well expressed in written and verbal work, of the problems a girl has when she has to explain her pregnancy to her parents, boy friend, head mistress. 'Phoebe' shows this in an imaginative way, the girl working out a variety of possible reactions to her news. On the other hand, this film was totally rejected by a group of biology teachers and a group of science teachers on training courses—it simply was not their medium. The Biology teachers preferred to use Thames Television's 'What's It All About?', where a boy and girl in London's dockland are faced with Phoebe's problem and where documentary generalization is used rather than imagination. More films need to be made about behavioural problems of the relations between the sexes using emotional identification, but this takes expertise in direction and acting. Most people with the required expertise can find more lucrative fields than that of educational films.

On the other hand, a set of loop films made by Eothen for use in Hertfordshire Youth Clubs are successful just because they do *not* invite identification. They present artificial, anonymous situations, which are common to the experience of adolescents, and which serve as 'Points of Departure' (the name of the series) for discussion on behavioural norms. They provide a firmer basis than

D

personal anecdote for such discussion as both discussion leader and class share the same visual experience and personal privacy does not have to be invaded. The loops are silent, the group is asked to provide a commentary, or to suggest what the characters are saying and thinking—a considerable exercise in non-verbal communication. The very artificiality of the situations provide laughter and consequently relaxed atmosphere for discussion; these loops have been very successfully used to structure, rather than to initiate, discussion in many schools and youth clubs throughout England and Wales.

Providing the extra-parental counsellor

Many people have been lucky 'o have such a counsellor readily available in an older sister, an uncle, a chemistry master at school, a mate in a job. In today's mobile society such counsellors are less likely to be available—teachers move more frequently, people change jobs more easily, housing planning has wrecked rather than encouraged social cohesiveness; lonely adolescents are common in urban life. Universities and the 'Underground' have recognized this need and for the intelligent 18- to 20-year-old facilities for advice and counselling on everything from landladies to VD are available and are used. For the rest, considerable tenacity and social expertise are needed to actually get oneself to a Brooks Centre (see page 59) (where counselling services are an obligatory part of contraceptive prescription) or to ask a youth or social worker the urgent questions. Many adolescents have been unused to asking questions on the subject and, if they dared to do so, have been given dusty, euphemistic or moralizing answers totally irrelevant to their situation; moreover, many find it difficult to make the counsellor aware of the whole range of attitudes and conditioning which make up the background to the question. Early education in vocabulary and communication skills, both social and verbal, are an essential prerequisite to successful counselling—otherwise an investigator rather than a counsellor is needed.

What is the role of the school in this matter? Some teachers are natural counsellors and whether they are designated so or not, pupils will go to them, learn from them and be supported by them. If any generalization can be made as to when to use neutrality and when to take a stand, it is that taking a stand is perhaps more used

74

in an individual counselling situation. But there is no simple answer here—the often quoted 'Give them the facts and let them make up their own minds' is a naive half-truth; it is better to give them the facts and the skills of the morally educated to help them to make rational decisions, while making sure that the pupils are also aware of the irrational factors which influence their behaviour, e.g. the basic drive to mating and parental behaviour, the effect of hormones.

Who then in the school can take on a counselling role? What really matters is the level of communication which the teacher has with the class, the degree of his knowledge about the attitudes, values and social mores of his pupils and that he knows the limits of knowledge or counselling which he can give. There will be pupils pathologically affected by sexual problems in all schools, and these are for the expert not the 'listening ear' type of counselling. School counsellors should be supported by such experts in case of need.

If a special counsellor is brought into the school, this will obviously remove much of the work from the general staff, but there will yet be those who prefer to take their troubles to the young History teacher, or the head, and the PE changing room is an ideal place for a quick, informal question. To be seen marching into the counsellor's office (or broom cupboard in one school!) may require face-saving explanations which may not be believed by one's fellows. The same may occur with counsellors in youth clubs, unless plenty of informal opportunities are provided for approaching the counsellor. One county provided a special counselling office in the middle of a shopping centre, but this required considerable nerve and determination for those in need of help actually to walk up the stairs. For such reasons, Croydon has begun an experiment with peripatetic counsellors going round the commercial coffee bars and discotheques, almost a domiciliary service. A telephone counselling service about VD is provided in Walsall, Bristol, Watford, Hitchin, Stirling and Glasgow, and many others are in the process of being organized, so great has been the demand on telephone services provided by VD clinics. The signs and symptoms of VD are given, plus the names and addresses of the clinics in the area, which are often repeated, or read out slowly so that they can be taken down, and Ansaphone-taped recordings are used to economize on staff.

In the class and small group counselling situation there will always be one or more adolescents who will not ask the questions they desperately need answering. They may not have accepted a counsellor, either formally or informally; they may not have the social courage to ask for an individual session. The way out for most girls here is to write to the women's magazines—they are totally confidential, whereas school teachers, counsellors, even social workers may not be. Boys, however, do not have this outlet, and, in general, lack both counselling opportunities and basic sex education[1], although there is a welcome change of opinion in many schools now. So provision must be made for the posing of anonymous questions, either by the use of a question box for written questions, or by providing a list of questions (such as are to be found in Schulz and Williams (1969), and the Gloucestershire Association for Family Life 2nd Report (1971)), and commenting on all, or asking the class to provide the answers, or by using the women's magazine correspondence columns for a group discussion of the questions and possible answers to compare with the advice given by the columnist.

A 13–14 group consisting of early maturing girls and late maturing boys may be totally unsuitable for such work, the girls may bully or embarrass the boys and vice versa. It takes an experienced teacher to ask why the little boys are sniggering; many, alas, just ignore the problem and battle on, with a consequent lack of communication education for all.

So what do the inexperienced do? First avoid any aspect of the subject towards which they feel an uncontrollable embarrassment. It is impossible to structure an unembarrassed class discussion when it is led by an embarrassed teacher. There is no shame involved in admitting to embarrassment, everyone has some aspect of sex and sexual behaviour which touches an emotional raw spot; those who have not must either be superhuman or subhuman! Secondly, to face up squarely to the sniggerers; they are sniggering basically

[1] Further, if we examine those children who learnt mainly from their peers, we find that 59·3 per cent of our older boys received only limited or no personal instruction in an area where no other type is satisfactory. 'That more than half our young men and one-third of our young women received their sex education from peer groups or the mass media must be alarming' (Ripley et al., 1971).

because they are embarrassed by open sex talk, and this is usually because they have been conditioned to think that sex is dirty. One teacher was quoted as saying, after his class had seen the BBC Merry-go-round programmes, 'There were only a few sniggers'. Perhaps it is idealistic to say that there should be none; sniggerers are vulnerable children in need of help. They lower the climate of discussion for the rest of the class, who, even today, are not absolutely sure that talking about sex is really the thing to do; the sniggerers renew their doubts. If the sniggering is obdurate, then social cohesiveness and a homogenous level of communication is impossible—the class must be divided into homogenous groups.

Finally, in whatever situation counselling takes place, it is necessary to examine as far as possible the reasons behind the asking of any question. Questions encouraged from the non-vocal section of the class by anonymous means, such as the use of a question box, preclude investigation into their origins—but if the questions are answered in class this may break down the barriers to communication and enable further inquiry either by pupil or teacher.

In some cases the answer is already in the questioner's mind and all that is needed is a 'listening ear' and supportive remarks. On the other hand, there may be a total inadequacy which needs counselling in some depth, or simply a need to show off some sexual prowess. Counselling is an emotionally demanding occupation and teachers who counsel in schools need to consider their own needs with respect to the emotional exhaustion which can ensue with excessive work in this field.

Professional courses for counsellors are provided at the Universities of Aston, Exeter, Keele, Swansea and Reading. Oxford, Wiltshire and Gloucestershire provide their own courses, but many other LEA's find it worthwhile to send teachers to the non-directive counselling courses run by the Marriage Guidance Council.

Education about marriage

Conceptually this is a vast and disorganized field, bravely tackled by the Marriage Guidance Council, the Catholic Marriage Advisory Council and the Jewish Marriage Council, all of whom have to divide their time and resources between repair of marital breakdown and preventive education. Recently, Social Studies syllabuses in schools have included the study of family life in depth in a variety of societies, choice of marriage partner and goals and expectations in marriage (see also page 42). Thus there has been a shift away from the emphasis on budgeting, furnishing your home and wedding etiquette (which used to figure so largely in school syllabuses) towards more fundamental concepts. The Duke of Edinburgh's Gold Awards Scheme includes an optional section on 'Getting married', where instruction is to be provided by Marriage Guidance Counsellors.

The BBC series 'The Family of Man' included some excellent comparisons between marriage as an institution in several different societies. Film is possibly the most effective method of structuring education about marriage for those who need it most; possibly the intelligent can deal with abstractions verbally, but for the majority visual education is accepted more readily and more easily retained. For the least able, few other methods are worth wasting time on. But even if film is used, it is difficult to fit the wide range of disciplines and experience which underly marriage education into a simple basic frame of reference and even more difficult to take account of individual variation. Is the objective total instruction over the whole field of psychosexual, physiological, cultural and social factors, or is it merely to make people aware of some of the factors involved? Can marriage education really do anything in the face of physical factors of attraction which lead so many adolescents to marry their opposites in philosophy of life and personality, with disastrous results? Some marriages of totally unlike people work well, so can anyone ever prescribe for anyone else in the matter of choice of marriage partner?

There is a case here for using the pathological as a means of education—Peter Dominian's *Marital Breakdown* (1968) is a very clearly written examination of factors involved and can certainly be used in sixth forms where perhaps it should be made required reading. Dominian advocates 'widespread education and preparation for marriage, the identification through research of its intrinsic destructive forces', many of which are concisely listed, with supporting evidence, in his book. It is not surprising that the younger people today have revolted from their elders' concepts of marriage, when they observe around them evidence of apathy and boredom, lack of communication (with husbands in the pub or at football, and wives at Bingo), and marriages only made tolerable by wife swapping or Bunny Club philosophies. Teachers dealing with man–woman roles and marriage styles in connection with the Humanities Project might find the Ciba symposium on *The Family and its Future* (1970) helpful. It is full of astringent remarks such as that of Robin Fox on family life, 'The failures are probably simply those families which refuse to ignore the natural conflicts inherent in the situation, while the successes are the families with the greatest capacity for collective self-delusion'.

Perhaps the most interesting provision of a simple frame of reference for thinking about marriage is that of Richard Hauser (Senior Research Fellow, Social Education and Social Planning) of Nottingham University. Students in training for teaching have benefitted from Hauser's ideas themselves and some have used his scheme with their pupils as a basis for the critical examination of marriage styles in films and novels.

Hauser proposes that there are five vital areas in marriage where the partners' ideas must either concur or where one partner agrees that the other's values must dominate and be accepted. If agreement is operational, rather than merely verbal, in three of these areas, Hauser postulates that the marriage will be viable and probably stable, whereas agreement in less than three indicates trouble. The areas are as follows:

1. *Sex.* If a nymphomaniac marries a homosexual agreement in this area is possible but unlikely. Lack of communication between partners on their position on the sexual continuum (often for reasons of guilt and shame felt by the individual because he or she does not fit into society's norms in this respect) can be seen in the letter columns of women's magazines. For example, the frequently occuring despair of a wife, whose husband and father of her children has just admitted that his homosexuality will not let him attempt to conform any longer. But even if agreement is reached on sexual matters before a partnership is entered into, there is no guarantee that the partner's needs will not change and develop with time.

2. *Family.* Are there still girls who prepare their layettes at the same time as they prepare their wedding dresses? Some girls

certainly see their partners as little else but the means towards fulfilling maternal drives. There are men who look on fatherhood merely as a proof that they can actually produce a child, while on the other hand some men are better at bringing up children than some women; fathers of one-parent families are often very successful as well as being heroic. Again, communication is important between partners, but this is often difficult because one partner may, at the conscious level, be willing to accept the values and attitudes of the other, but may be lacking in the self-knowledge to realize that for them such acquiescence is impossible.

3. *Tenderness*. To many women this is an essential part of the partnership and some will go to any lengths to ensure at least a superficial display, such as remembered anniversaries and frequent gifts of flowers; one wife actually bought an Easter egg for her own husband to give to her. On the other hand, there are women to whom this means little and when given a bunch of flowers are likely to wonder what sin had prompted the gift. Touch taboos operate in some British sub-cultures, others equate tenderness with softness. Agreement here is essential.

4. *Partnership*. For some, total involvement with each other's work and leisure is essential. For example, in creative artists who may wish to spend 24 hours per day, seven days per week, with each other, although in all truth this is difficult to maintain for a twenty-year period. For others, for example, Army officers and much-travelled business men, a wife has to be someone who can get on without very much partnership. Many feel that they must conform to society's views in the matter and it is pathetic to see husbands with bright smiles helping with their wives' favourite charity fete and wives grimly pretending to enjoy golf. The ever-present letters from wives who have guilt feelings because they even dare to think about holidays apart from their husbands still occur in correspondence columns.

5. *Values*. The conflict of the idealistic wife who has a totally materialistic husband has been exploited in plays, novels and films. The difficulties of Catholic marrying Jew, of gipsy marrying suburbanite are obvious. This is the most important aspect of all and since it is the one which requires most abstract thought and is

often confused by long conditioned emotion, it is perhaps the most difficult area for compromise.

All in all, Hauser's simple analysis says that one must decide who one is, and where one is going before deciding who one is going with. Nevertheless, the most rational being is still likely to be confounded by 'nature's gigantic plot', the well disguised attributes of Eros as opposed to Agape.

Education in the emotional and communicative aspects of parental roles

Henry Mayhew's 'Those who will not work' (1862) describes the promiscuous behaviour of 'female operatives' (shop girls, milliners) and maid-servants and attributes it to several causes, among which is the 'Absence of parental care and inculcation of proper precepts. In short, bad bringing up'.

This concept has been too often superficially ascribed to 'broken homes' and delinquent parents, but this example from Tunnadine's work (1970) shows the true nature of this factor. She describes a trendy girl who had had her first baby at 15, and came to a family planning clinic 'because she thought she ought to go on the pill' after an abortion at 19. It is this kind of behaviour which provokes outraged cries against the 'permissive' way of life from those who only perceive such matters superficially—but Tunnadine investigated further and found that for this girl 'intercourse had been nothing. At home they were only happy if she was out of the way. Her fruitless quest from stranger to stranger was for the love and tenderness she had never known at home'.

Teachers and social workers at least will recognize a common collection of characteristics possessed by Mayhew's ladies and Tunnadine's girl, over 100 years later; Mayhew held up his hands in horror, as many do today; Tunnadine's girl responded to counselling and while it is unlikely that she lived happily ever after, her life took a less erratic and more satisfying course afterwards, as she improved her relationships with other humans, including her parents.

Too often this kind of behaviour is part of a vicious circle which begins with an unwanted child, whether within or outside marriage, or with a child whose parents have no knowledge of its emotional and mental needs and devote themselves only to the physical and material aspects of child care; love is expressed as an excess of sweets or a new tape recorder, but in no other way. With puberty and the search for a secure adult identity, such children are very vulnerable to a variety of social influences.

At adolescence, boys may use aggression as a substitute for their frustrated need of genuine affection and consideration at home—and this includes aggression against self through the use of hard drugs. Girls looking for a substitute may accept the bonding caused by sexual attraction in place of love—how can they know what love is since they have never received it? They may enjoy flaunting their new-found sexuality not only to receive admiration but also to demonstrate how adult they are, how ready to escape from their unpleasant childhood bondage and be free to make their own friends and enjoy themselves. All these factors can lead to so-called promiscuity, and abortion, illegitimacy or VD. If it leads to illegitimacy in most cases it will close the circle. The mother who has never had the security of knowing that she is loved and lovable often has little idea of a genuinely considerate mother's role (see diagram on pages 88–9).

Some psychosexual experts think that getting pregnant, in spite of knowing how not to, is a call for attention, possibly of the man the girl hopes to marry; but pregnancy will bring the attention of the social services at least, if nothing else. Other girls have said that they wanted the baby because it would be something of their own, something which would have to pay them attention, or a defence against loneliness. Others use their abortions or VD treatment as a means of getting attention, and talk with bravado to anyone who will listen about the number of times they have been cured. Such girls are often quoted as examples of the way sex education encourages sexual licence; but any sex education they may have had assumes that they are rational beings, which by the frustration of their most basic need, to be respected by themselves and by others (which includes being loved and being able to love) they cannot be. Such a life history is described with great emotional impact in the film 'Gale is Dead' (BBC, now from Concord Films), which shows a girl going from institution to institution, with a variety of foster homes and help from well-meaning people who could not supply what she was looking for, and finally ending in death from heroin. Narrow sex education cannot help such girls, but education in parental roles may help to break the vicious circle. There are no statistics to show that boys who have been unable to identify with a parental role, whose fathers have been remote or died when the boy was young, or have been removed by divorce, themselves become poor fathers, but it is thought that, for example, orphanage children are particularly at risk and divorced parents are counselled on this danger to their child's development. Some of the factors involved in this situation for both sexes are shown in the diagram, but these are only a few of the factors involved.

The most developed work in this field is that of Mrs. Jane Madders, who was until recently lecturer in Health and Social Science at the City of Birmingham College of Education. Mrs. Madders realized that those in most need of education in parental roles are also those who are poor at learning abstractions, possibly lack reading skills and needed to learn by experiencing situations with children under guidance and with discussion. She made it possible for 14-year-old 'difficult' girls to be released from school to act as assistants in nursery and play groups where they could deal with children, feeding them, learning about nutrition, talking to them, learning how a child communicates at various ages, playing with them, seeing how play helps a child to grow mentally and socially, reading stories to them and so improving their own reading skills. Mrs. Madders and her colleagues used such situations for *ad hoc* teaching on some fairly abstract concepts such as physical and mental development, including language and spatial concepts and, above all, the ways of fulfilling a child's needs for security of affection. The girls may also go home with the mothers of these children to learn from the home situation and compare the child's behaviour there with his behaviour in the play group.

It is impossible to evaluate such work. All that can be said is that the girls are interested in it and even the most hardened school-haters enjoy it, and not merely as an escape from the classroom. (This in contrast to the traditional classes in child care rejected by London schoolgirls who said they had enough of that sort of thing at home.) It remains to be seen whether these girls will overcome years of conditioning and adopt more productive attitudes when

83

bringing up their own children. A film of her work with these girls was made by Mrs. Madders and is available from her. In at least one area in the country similar work has been done with boys, only in this case the overt objective was for the boys to consolidate their science by going into primary schools, teaching simple investigatory work and in so doing learning how to communicate with children of this age group and to understand their difficulties. With the increasing fluidity of sex roles in this country at the moment, boys in Oxford have worked in play groups, while in the Denaby Main Experiment (New Society, September 1971) boys cooked the play-group's lunches.

Physical and material aspects of parental roles

Descriptions of milestones of development during the first five years of a child's life appear frequently in women's magazines, and some schools teach this work also. The Croydon Health Education Department has successfully used the films of the National Film Board of Canada series, 'Ages and Stages', which were made in the 1950's and are still relevant today; this series also deals with emotional development from the early years to adolescence. A full description of methods and media will be found in *Health Education —Patterns for Teaching*, a resource collection for use in schools and health education work with other groups (Elliott and May, 1969).

Pat Parrish of the Carshalton Health Education Centre describes her work in one aspect of this field as follows:

It is rather encouraging to note that boys and girls think of marriage as equal partnership. To help them work out the ways in which duties and responsibilities are shared in the home, I use a flannel graph to assist discussion, with a man on one side and a woman on the other, placing under them various symbols representing their contributions to family life. Who earns the money? In many cases these days both father and mother do. Who looks after the baby? Usually Mum, but father helps sometimes even with the midnight feed. Who actually pays the bills? In the working class home the father may hand over all or most of his pay packet to Mum who does the paying, but in middle class homes father usually pays all. Who does the decorating, gardening, letter writing? By this time the majority of the duties have landed in the column headed by the woman. However, it is cheering to note that a new generation of co-operative fathers has arisen.

It is interesting to note that today's young men in their twenties seem to have more security of self-image than their fathers had and do not worry about losing face when doing traditionally feminine duties such as nappy changing—and this in spite of the fact that few of them would ever have benefitted from the education provided by the Humanities Project or the Moral Education Project in such matters. They have adopted the considerate way of life unaided. So it seems that such education may indeed have a chance of overcoming years of conditioning and the effect of social and cultural pressures, in some of our sub-cultures at least.

Education about venereal diseases

In their survey on 'Sex attitudes of young people' (Holmes *et al.*, 1968) it was found that only 23 per cent of a control group (matched with young patients attending a VD clinic) had any knowledge about VD. In Granada TV's follow-up of their series of sex education programmes 'Understanding' (1967) 32 per cent of school children in their middle teens said that they had no knowledge at all of the facts about VD which were presented; this was the programme in the series most preferred by the pupils. A health educator working with recruits to the Women's Services (1971) reports wide ignorance in this field. Meanwhile, although overall VD rates are going down, rates for adolescents are on the increase; the much-used American film on the subject 'One Quarter of a Million Teenagers' is now re-titled 'Half a Million Teenagers', showing a similar trend in the USA.

Glass, Atkinson and Rickett (1968) showed that even those teaching about VD had some surprising gaps in their knowledge. Their paper 'What do the educated know about VD?' includes the questionnaire they used to diagnose lack of knowledge in a way which allowed people to admit ignorance without losing face. Similar pre-test techniques have been used in this country with school children, student and in-service teachers. The University of Melbourne has produced an audio-tutorial programme for in-service teacher training on VD.

While the need to remedy such widespread ignorance is apparent, several health educators are of the opinion that VD should be seen as yet another infectious disease rather than in a context of its own; this is also the view of the Nuffield Secondary Science Project (1971) in *Theme 3—The Biology of Man*, where VD is treated at the end of the section on 'Health and hygiene'.

The Schools Council Humanities Project includes one sheet giving a concise appraisal of the statistics of the situation and dispelling the myth that immigrants are responsible for the increase in VD in the UK. (Since the excerpt comes from the *Morning Star*, capitalist society comes in for a major share of the blame). In the Schools Council Moral Education Project, VD is not mentioned specifically, but in the 'Consequences' section of the material, classes are asked to discuss what might happen as a result of various actions, one of which (48) is 'sleeps with casual acquaintances' and another (77) 'moves about as usual when he has an infectious illness'.

In Sheffield, parents consulted by the local health education service generally agreed that they would prefer to have the basic facts about VD given to their children at the age of 12 or 13 before many of them are at risk or too emotionally involved to be able to think clearly on the subject. On display at the Sheffield Health Education Centre is a permanent and comprehensive exhibition on VD which has been used with schools, youth clubs, and adult organizations including parents. Only when it was loaned to a university project did it attract the attention of graffiti. Sheffield's programme has been running since 1960 and while it is difficult to evaluate its effects on the epidemiological pattern, there is general agreement that it has contributed to more open attitudes on the subject and has increased the willingness of those at risk to come forward for examination and treatment.

So the objectives of VD education are at least twofold, including not only the provision of the basic facts but also producing a social climate where, for example, girls with a vaginal discharge due to a fungus (Monilia sp.) can go to a clinic without shame rather than write a despairing letter to a women's magazine. These objectives are perhaps easily achieved with the intelligent and the literate, for example, by the use of the material in the Schools Council General

Studies Project, or by reading the various paperback books on the subject. A South London School approaches the problem through literature, using Frances Brett Young's *House under the Water* and *Portnoy's Complaint*. The BBC has produced excellent programmes on VD, but it is doubtful that those in most need of such education ever see them. The Health Education Council's posters, such as 'How to catch gonorrhoea', offended many people by their forthrightness, but at least made some attempt to reach the most important target population for VD education. In one area in the north, the LHA showed films about VD in the cafes most frequented by prostitutes.

Educating teachers

The scheme of *Education in Personal Relationships* drawn up by a working party of teachers from the City of Exeter (Exeter Education Committee, 1970) considers that the four main elements in in-service teacher training for this work are:

'1. Methods of securing and maintaining parental co-operation.

2. Factual medical information on (a) the mental and physical development of children, and (b) human reproduction.

3. Discussion of attitudes towards ethical and moral issues and preparation of parenthood.

4. Practical advice on classroom techniques and visual aids.'

The working party recommends co-operation with the school health department and the child guidance centre when dealing with section 2, and with moral welfare and marriage guidance organizations when dealing with section 3. For section 4, 'A short demonstration course given under classroom conditions can often achieve far more than formal discussions'; while this may be true, nevertheless the artificial situation created by any demonstration lesson could be undesirable, especially as in this case the teacher might be visiting an unfamiliar class which would add problems of communication and lack of knowledge of individual needs and attitudes.

Video-tape recording of lessons by teachers with their own classes is being used to overcome these difficulties; for example, the Audio-Visual Centre of the University of York has produced a programme where a tutor traces a lesson on reproduction in mammals using

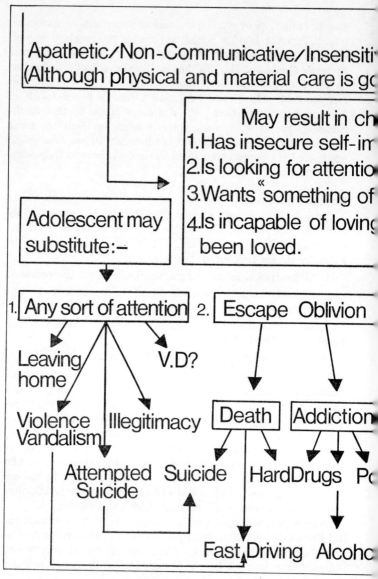

Apathetic/Non-Communicative/Insensiti
(Although physical and material care is go

May result in ch
1. Has insecure self-im
2. Is looking for attentio
3. Wants "something of
4. Is incapable of loving
been loved.

Adolescent may substitute:–

1. Any sort of attention   2. Escape Oblivion

Leaving home   V.D?

Violence Vandalism   Illegitimacy   Death   Addiction

Attempted Suicide   Suicide   HardDrugs   P

Fast Driving   Alcoho

88

PARENTAL CARE

which:—

.

t least, if not love.

own."

it has never

Lacks concepts of parental roles

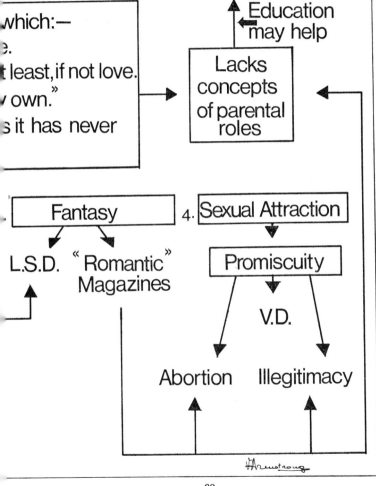

Education may help

Fantasy

4. Sexual Attraction

L.S.D. "Romantic" Magazines

Promiscuity

V.D.

Abortion   Illegitimacy

H.Armstrong

video-tape inserts of a class of 12-year-old grammar school pupils dissecting pregnant mice in a Nuffield 'O' Level Biology situation.

The Mobile Recording Unit of the Faculty of Education, King's College, London, has taped three different types of lessons in sex education, using remote-controlled, very small and unobtrusive pillar cameras which do little to disrupt the well-established communications between the teacher and the class. One of these is on the use of the Nuffield Resources for Learning Projects' programmed learning on the basic facts of human reproduction for non-streamed 11-year-olds in a large comprehensive school. The second is of a wide-ranging discussion with an English teacher and a group of Jamaican and English girls (including one Cypriot), in a very non-academic class of 14-year-olds in London; the teacher weaves a difficult middle way between too much control of the ebullient discussion and a threatened take-over by those with the loudest voices.

The third tape is of a CSE class in English, working on a theme 'Ain't love grand!' showing one lesson of a piece of work which extended over several weeks. The girls bought in articles, photographs and poems on the theme, discussed and commented on them, and made a wall display of their own writing, pictures and excerpts from a wide variety of sources, including women's magazines, William Blake and the marriage service.

Thus these three tapes show three very different approaches, but equally important ones.

The King's College Mobile Recording Unit has also made videotapes of teacher in-service and initial training for use with international visitors interested in this field. The factual needs of mature teachers vary enormously and several authorities are examining the possibilities of resources centres with an individual programming approach where, for example, a man teacher, aware of his deficiencies in both fact and concept when teaching about birth, can use a programme of video-tape, film, books and slides to fill in the gaps. This would be followed by an individual tutorial—since no programme is ever entirely suited to the needs of every individual.

Nor can teachers entirely rely on others for the selection of visual aids for their classes (see section on visual symbolism). This provides a real problem of time in in-service courses, as ideally every teacher needs to see the vast variety of visual aids, particularly films, which are available and select those appropriate for his own class, taking into account their mental age, level of understanding and cultural backgrounds, as well as their emotional maturity. Teachers are busy people; the Grampian series on 'Living and Growing' has shown that the greater proportion of both teachers and parents prefer a preview of programmes to be in the comfort of their own homes—and this would seem a useful solution to the problem of film viewing, if either BBC or ITA were prepared to take up the work involved. At present there is much duplication by local authority panels, science teachers and health educators on film evaluation and no central co-ordination of the results.

With the initial training of teachers both in colleges and departments of education similar problems present themselves, but in addition there is the basic problem of how students can fill in their factual gaps without losing face before their peers. Many colleges use team-teaching; for example, the Centre for Science Education at Chelsea College organized each year two inter-collegiate team-teaching sessions for all science graduates training for teaching the London area. These sessions were supported by previous preparation, possibly using seminars and films, in the various colleges and also followed up. The sessions themselves deal mainly with the problems and methods of sex education, the necessary integration of moral education (based on the Wilson criteria) with biological fact and the extension of the usual interpretation of 'sex education' to cover the whole of the human life cycle. The sessions used visiting experts, both in the general introductory sessions and in group discussions; these experts have included experienced teachers, journalists, a TV director, National Childbirth Trust and IPPF officials and a very successful VD social worker. Such co-ordination is efficient in the use of experts' time—there are relatively few of these people about, and many of them waste too much time and energy travelling to small groups around the country.

What is often missing or not made explicit rather than implicit in teacher training courses is work on the psychological aspects of sexual behaviour such as ambivalence, aggression and transference, as John Wilson has pointed out (private communication). General psychology courses touch on these matters, but on the whole leave the student with no clear frame of reference with which to work when dealing with pupils' problems.

Several authorities select their teachers for work in this field, according to recommendation from heads and their behaviour on a residential course where they are helped to evaluate their own degree of psychological freedom in sexual matters. On the whole, however, teachers select themselves.[1] What is needed is for those who are genuinely embarrassed by discussing sex with pupils but feel obliged to do so by their own sense of duty should be helped to realize that such self-immolation is neither necessary nor desirable. At the other end of the scale, there is the obsessed teacher who uses his classes as his own private *News of the World*.

A variety of teachers, young and old, mature and immature, demonstrating a variety of attitudes, methods and roles, both communicative, informative and authoritative, provides the ideal situation for sex education in its widest sense rather than searching for any one ideal teacher.

References

CIBA FOUNDATION SYMPOSIUM (1970). *The Family and Its Future*. London: Churchill.

DOMINIAN, P. (1968). *Marital Breakdown*. London: Penguin.

DUKE OF EDINBURGH'S AWARD SCHEME. Information from 2, Old Queen Street, London SW1.

ELLIOTT, D. and MAY, E. (1969). *Health Education: Patterns for Teaching*. London: Macmillan.

EXETER EDUCATION COMMITTEE (1970). *Scheme of Education in Personal Relationships*, from City Education Office, 33, St. David's Hill, Exeter, EX4 4DE. 5p.

GLASS, L., ATKISSON, L. and RICKETT, M. (1968). 'What do the educated know about VD?' *Internat. J. Health*, 3rd quarter. USA.

GLOUCESTERSHIRE ASSOCIATION FOR FAMILY LIFE (1966). *Education for Personal Relationships and Family Life*. Second Annual Report. Now out of print.

HOLMES, M., NICOL, C. and STUBBS, R. (1968). 'Sex attitudes of young people.' *Educ. Res.*, **11,** 1, 38–42.

[1] This is obviously a subjective assessment but it does seem to have worked effectively and generally avoids the difficult situation of failing or excluding teachers (Lewis, 1970).

LEWIS, D. (1970). *Sex Education in Secondary Schools*. Duplicated copies from Health Education Adviser, City of Oxford Education Committee, PO Box 24, City Chambers, Queen Street, Oxford.

MAYHEW, H. (1862). 'Those who will not work.' In: QUENNELL, P. (ed.) (1950). *London's Underworld*. London: Spring Books.

MORRIS, D. (1967). *The Naked Ape*. London: Galaxy.

NUFFIELD SECONDARY SCIENCE PROJECT (1971). *Theme 3—The Biology of Man*. London: Longmans.

RIPLEY, G. D., BURNS, C. and DICKINSON, V. A. (1971). 'A survey of sexual knowledge and attitudes in Borehamwood.' *The Practitioner*. September, 207.

SCHOOLS COUNCIL GENERAL STUDIES PROJECT (1972). Information from The Secretary, General Studies Project, The King's Manor, York.

SCHULZ, E. and WILLIAMS, S. (1969). *Family Life and Sex Education: Curriculum and Instruction*. USA: Harcourt, Brace & World Inc.

TUNNADINE, L. P. D. (1970). *Contraception and Sexual Life*. London: Tavistock.

Films

BRITISH BROADCASTING CORPORATION: 'Family of Man.' TV programme, available for hire in black and white, from BBC TV Enterprises Film Hire, 25, The Burroughs, Hendon, London NW4. £5 each.

BRITISH BROADCASTING CORPORATION: 'Gale is Dead.' From Concord Films, Nacton, Ipswich.

BOULTON-HAWKER. 'Barnet—The Child,' from Foundation Film Library, Brooklands House, Weybridge, Surrey.

BOULTON-HAWKER. 'Half a Million Teenagers,' from Foundation Film Library, Brooklands House, Weybridge, Surrey.

COLES, M. 'Growing Up,' from Global Films, 143, Wardour Street, London W1. Hire charge £8, including postage.

EOTHEN. 'Learning to Live,' from Sound Services, 269, Kingston Road, London SW19.

EOTHEN. 'Points of Departure.' Series of film loops, from Sound Services, 269, Kingston Road, London SW19.

EOTHEN. 'To Janet a Son?' From Farleys Goods, Galleymead Road, Colnbrook, Bucks.

MADDERS, J. Film of Assisting in Play Groups. From 6, Selly Close, Selly Wick Road, Birmingham 29.

NATIONAL FILM BOARD OF CANADA. 'Phoebe.' From Concord Films, Nacton, Ipswich.

SCHOOLS COUNCIL HUMANITIES PROJECT. 'Sex is Everywhere.' From Associated British Pathe, Film House, 142, Wardour Street, London W1.

THAMES TELEVISION. 'What's It All About?' Inquiries to Thames TV, 306, Euston Road, London, NW1 3BB.

CHAPTER FIVE

Evaluation in Sex Education

IN SEX EDUCATION, invasion of personal privacy means that evaluation can be very difficult, if not impossible. Sometimes the criteria of an evaluation are merely that the work did not upset the children, teachers or parents or school governors, and while this is important it is obvious that more research in depth is needed. And how is one to evaluate the teaching and learning of the Wilsonian criteria? The multitude of variables involved in moral education and the expense of long-term investigation into attitude changes make such work rare, although Wilson has himself devised some assessment instruments, and Stenhouse is engaged on long-term attitude testing. Examples chosen, therefore, represent a wide range of evaluation procedures from the purely subjective to Roger's more sophisticated approach; each in its own way is valuable, each has its own drawbacks.

One of the most amusing evaluation studies (on sex education textbooks) is 'Sex Education: the erroneous zone' (Hill and Jones, 1970). This pamphlet points out the idiocies of many such recommended works for adolescents and causes speculation as to whether teachers can actually have read these books before passing them on to their unsuspecting classes. 'The sperm . . . are very pleased indeed to find themselves right at the top of the vaginal passage', is one gem, closely followed by 'The losing sperm in the race all perish, which is their punishment for failing to reach what might have been their destiny'. Such books, pilloried by these authors, must have caused a good deal of anxiety to a generation of adolescents. Moreover, as the authors point out, 'They are not likely to listen to advice from people who will not be honest with them', but the authority of the printed word is such that many will have accepted it and suffered because of it. Here at least the working class child is at an advantage—he doesn't read long-winded books, such as those on the Hill and Lloyd Jones' list, but the middle class child, whose sex education used to come largely from such books, has been seriously at risk.

Direct opinion evaluation in a boys' school

In a London boys' school, the basic communications and facts of sex are taught by the Biology department in the fourth form in rather more detail than the 'O' level syllabus requires. VD, abortion, and boy/girl relationships are included. In 1971 the staff gave the 52 boys involved an unannounced questionnaire, which they completed within about 15 minutes. Thirty-nine boys thought that giving information on sex to the fourth form was necessary—others thought that it should be given in the second or third forms and four said it was unnecessary; further questions showed that these four boys had had information from books, friends and parents. Some gave the source of their information as being dirty jokes, over half had had information from friends and books and less than half from parents.

When they were asked what they had learned in the Biology lessons which they had not known before, birth, menstruation and VD were mentioned. In a question asking for brief definitions of various terms, those who had answered that they had learned nothing new in their Biology lessons feature prominently among those who gave unsatisfactory answers; there's none so ignorant as those who don't know that they don't know—or is it that it involves loss of face to admit ignorance even to a questionnaire?

'Did you find any of the information given in the Biology lessons distasteful?' 'Yes', said one boy. 'Masturbation. It should be left to the boy, he doesn't need telling. Too personal for school.' 'No', said all but two. 'I don't think anything about sex is distasteful. It is necessary to learn about it. (Maybe VD is distasteful.) Nothing should be left unmentioned'. Some boys asked for work on prostitution and on the moral side of sex and marriage to be included.

But the same question was asked by these intelligent middle class boys as in Alan Harris's secondary modern class (see Harris, 1970), and which appears in any question box used in a sex education lesson: adolescents really want to know what all the fuss about intercourse is due to. This, as shown by the Hill and Lloyd Jones' (1970) survey is what few books for adolescents describe, except in a purely mechanical way. (Methods of teaching about the experience of intercourse will be found on page 68.)

If more simple evaluations of this kind had taken place we would not be faced today with Schofield's finding that many adolescents who were interviewed by him five years ago and said that they had had sex education have by now changed their minds and realized that they had not had anything like the amount they needed.

The revised Schofield study

In 1955 Michael Schofield, then the Research Director of the Central Council for Health Education, investigated a carefully selected sample of young people. Using pre-tested interview schedules he evaluated the extent of teenage activities and attitudes towards sex and examined the difference between the sexually experienced teenager and others (Schofield, 1972).

This study revealed the lack of sex education among teenagers, and in particular those who were sexually experienced had had less sex education than the others. Schofield has now asked similar questions of the same people seven years later, and the full results of his survey will be published by the Health Education Council in 1972. The new figures indicate that those who said that they had had sex education in 1965 had changed their minds by 1970, and when asked (by now in their early twenties) if they felt that they knew all they needed to know, 40 per cent of the boys and 31 per cent of the girls said 'No'. Of those who still agreed that they had had sex education, many said that it was too late, and did not tell them what they wanted to know, such as more about the physical make-up of the opposite sex. Eighty per cent would have liked more sex education at school; 64 per cent learned about sex from their peers, but only two per cent thought that this was a good method. Sixty per cent would have preferred more information from their parents.

This all adds up to a miserable picture of inadequacy and points up the fact that the widening of the concept of sex education from the purely anatomical and physiological to take in the behavioural, emotional and moral aspects is long overdue. The full report, *Sexual Development*, will be published by the Health Education Council in the Spring of 1972.

Feedback in curriculum development: the Nuffield Secondary Science Project (13-16)

The Schools Council's Working Paper No. 1 (1964, now out of print) sets out the basic brief of the Nuffield Secondary Science Project's work on the human life cycle, growth and development. It was assumed that much of the work could be based on previous knowledge of animal life cycles and of simple human anatomy and physiology, including pubertal changes. After initial trials (1967) of this section in schools it became obvious that this work had not always been dealt with before 13-plus and would need to be added to the text. Apart from this and the exclusion of recommended work on the homologies of the male and female reproductive organs, the original outline held good.

Both verbal and written feedback from teachers indicated that some guidance as to the nature of morality was needed and so Wilson's criteria for moral education (see page 28) were included and appear in the introduction to this section, giving examples of particular pieces of work where they could be used as a basic objective. Some teachers felt that 12-plus was a little early for discussion on morals and preferred to leave an ethical approach until later in the course. However, the need for moral judgements crept in when schools used a series of slides showing human embryos; when several classes raised the problem of the ethics of photographing dead babies. It is noteworthy that the same questions arose, according to a Swedish inspector, when pupils in the north of Sweden saw the film 'Barnet'; they were distressed at seeing still photographs of human embryos, in colour, which seemed even more still in a film where everything else moved.

Teachers in the trials of the material were asked to say where they felt they needed additional sources of information because their knowledge of a topic was limited. Examples of such topics requested and now included in the published material were interpretive diagrams of the human-embryos slides and of two X-rays showing a foetus *in utero*. It must be remembered that many of the teachers concerned were not biology specialists. Extensive references were included; for example, Dalton (1970). References to some pamphlets were deleted as the feedback indicated that the boys and girls judged them to be 'too childish'. Teachers commented on the lack of suitable reading material on sex for the less proficient readers, who nevertheless demand adult treatment in such texts and possibly a strip cartoon approach.

The background knowledge of the classes varied widely, as did their attitudes. In some schools the discussion of sexual matters was difficult and the boys and girls showed some embarrassment; 13 is often too late to change attitudes ingrained after long conditioning. On the whole, however, both parents and pupils appreciated the work.

The pupils generally felt a sense of relief that questions about sexual behaviour could be and were discussed. In some schools the integrated approach recommended in the text had been used to advantage in team teaching situations with English and Humanities specialists. At the other end of the life cycle, consideration for the life of the aged made such an impact in one school that the pupils decided things must change radically before they themselves grew old.

As expected, there was great variation in evaluations of the various visual aids recommended. Cassettes were preferred because of the difficulties of obtaining a 16mm film exactly when it was needed. The most used cassettes were those produced by Eothen films ('Man and Woman' Parts I and II, and 'Childbirth'), showing diagrammatically menstruation, intercourse and childbirth. Teachers, however, were critical of their defects; in 'Man and Woman I' the egg disappears before fertilization in the uterus as if by magic, while in 'Man and Woman II' fertilization occurs before copulation and one class thought that fertilization therefore occurred in some other way (see also page 68). The wide choice of other films recommended meant that further generalization was difficult or impossible. Those teachers who did use the Eothen 'Points of Departure' series of loop films agreed that they were useful in helping to structure discussion on adolescent behaviour (see also page 73).

While it is true to say that the Nuffield Secondary Science material initiated discussion in some schools on the advisability and structuring of a course on sex education, most of the teachers in the non-selective schools concerned with the project already had some form of curriculum in this field. What Secondary Science did for the majority was to provide resources needed, both of authority and material.

Evaluations of two showings of Grampian TV's 'Living and Growing' in 1968 and 1970

Grampian describes itself as a 'fairly small member of ITV' and hence unable to embark on a major evaluation programme with respect to these transmissions. Nevertheless, comparisons between the 1968 and 1970 figures, obtained from teachers' reports, are interesting, and deserve a total appraisal rather than the selection of a few parameters which is all that space permits here.

	1968	1970	
Number of Reports from teachers	148	136	
Number of children whose reactions were reported	3,800	5,500	
Number of teachers who had not previously included human reproduction in the syllabus	72%	62%	
Percentage of teachers who had seen previews	45%	35% (seen previous transmission)	
Who had watched evening series for adults	80%	80%	
Used programme notes	85%	77%	

The fact that so many schools were able to include human reproduction in their work which had not done so previously says much for the way in which the programmes were introduced to parents and teachers as well as being a compliment to their overall design. There is also the factor of the powerful authority of such TV programmes in changing attitudes. Grampian added to this authority and the acceptability of the programmes by using a doctor as the presenter.

Secondly, these figures indicate that both teachers and parents prefer their training to be at home rather than at meetings outside it. This is largely due to people having a strenuous working day, and indicates an understandable unwillingness to leave home comforts for school meetings. Possibly it might also imply that parents would rather discuss such matters privately than in public, as well as the fact that television captures a large audience through the inability to switch off late in the evenings.

From the pupil's point of view, although their reactions are necessarily filtered through the teachers, the opening up of communications between them and their parents seems to have been very welcome. One 11-year-old girl said 'I did not discuss this at home before we got the programmes' and a 13-year-old said 'My mother has been watching the programmes as well—I don't feel so embarrassed to ask her things I wouldn't have asked before'.

Reactions to the programmes themselves were as follows.

Programme:

1. General introduction, the life cycle and the family.	Both boys and girls knew most of the information and this programme raised little comment from half the children.
2. Heredity and parental contributions.	Few knew much about the facts here and much discussion was provoked.
3. Basic biological facts of puberty.	About a third knew their facts here—the break-through here was on communication. 'There was a deathly silence after the programme in which the actual word 'penis' was used, but practically without exception embarrassment was short-lived and sensible relevant discussion followed'.
4. Menstruation.	Boys were very ignorant here, but it was the girls who discussed it most, both in 1968 and 1970—illustrating that the facts are not enough—it is their application to the individual which matters.
5. Gestation.	This was the area showing highest ignorance in both transmissions.

6. Birth.	Again a fairly high level of ignorance.
7. Discussion on previous programme.	Since so much discussion had already taken place in class, this programme was considered a waste of time by some teachers.
8. Living and growing as a cycle. Consolidation of previous programmes.	Although in both transmissions pupils knew most of the facts, two-thirds were still interested in discussing it, illustrating the need for consolidation and reinforcement in sex education as well as in other parts of the curriculum (see also pages 37 and 102).

Pre-testing and post-testing in sex education

Evaluation, as the previous examples have shown, is usually at the end of a course of instruction and rarely measures changes in knowledge acquired. Often information comes from the pupils via the teacher; even a questionnaire given by the teacher is likely to influence the answers given. There have also been surveys on young peoples' attitudes to sex; for example, that of Dr. Robert Kind (1969), and of the Gloucestershire Association for Family Life (1966). Rarely, however, has there been any investigation into change of attitude and knowledge as a result of sex education, which is why the work of the Communication and Attitude Change Research Unit at LSE is welcome in this field.

The unit, not unnaturally, found that tests of sexual knowledge and attitude appropriate to the age group eight to ten, for which the BBC Merry-go-round programmes were intended, were non-existent and they carefully structured their own. They used the schools where the BBC pilot broadcasts had been made to try out the effectiveness of their tests which were free essays and tests of specific knowledge gained. Parents were also questioned, teachers gave an assessment of the ability range of the classes and an observer in the classroom during the follow-up discussion of each programme (which his presence might well have inhibited) recorded children's questions.

Preliminary evidence (Rogers, 1971) indicates that knowledge was gained without emotional distress and that concepts about growing up changed from generalizations to specific factors, while concepts on birth shifted away from the idea of birth as an operation. This evidence indicates that sex education in the primary school can help to promote a more healthy acceptance of natural bodily functions. Parental approval of the programmes increased after they were shown—this feature is also noted in the survey of opinions on the showing of Grampian's 'Living and Growing' series as well as in many American studies. In the Grampian survey (Gill *et al.*, 1971), 77 per cent of those who had not seen any of the 'Living and Growing' series supported the idea that such education was necessary and the number in favour increased to 85 per cent of those who had seen the programmes.

Those interested in research might start thinking about how they could possibly evaluate the achievement of the variety of objectives named below, which provide a consensus from many sources.

1. To impart a thorough understanding of the human life cycle.

2. To remove ignorance and fear of sexual matters by providing the necessary information.

3. To promote the considerate way of life, particularly in sexual matters, which have great potentiality for the causation of human misery.

4. To help each individual to accept, improve or adjust his potentialities as a human being as well as a sexual person, rather than conforming to norms imposed by others, in so far as this is compatible with the considerate life style.

5. To enable individuals to make responsible decisions about their own personal lives, while realizing that many choices in this field are irrational.

6. To promote an acceptable climate of discussion between men and women, boys and girls, parents and children, so that sex education in its widest sense can begin where it should, at an early age and in the home.

References

DALTON, K. (1970). *The Menstrual Cycle*. London: Penguin.

GILL, D., REID, G. and SMITH, D. (1971). 'Sex education, press and parental perceptions.' *The Health Educ. J.*, **30**, 1.

GLOUCESTERSHIRE ASSOCIATION FOR FAMILY LIFE (1966). *Attitudes to Religious Health and Sex Education. The Attitudes of Young People*. Loan copies available from GAFL, 2, College Street, Gloucester.

GRAMPIAN TV (1968). 'Living and Growing.' *A Report on a Sex Education Series for Primary Schools*. From Queen's Cross, Aberdeen, AB9 2XJ.

HARRIS, A. (1970). *Thinking About Education*. London: Heinemann.

HILL, M. and LLOYD JONES, M. (1970). *Sex Education: the erroneous zone*. From National Secular Society, 103, Borough High Street, London SE1.

KIND, R. (1969). 'The sexual attitudes of young people.' *Family Planning*, **18**, 1.

NUFFIELD SECONDARY SCIENCE PROJECT. *Theme 3—The Biology of Man*. London: Longmans.

ROGERS, R. (1971). 'The effects of sex education.' *New Society*. 3rd June.

SCHOFIELD, M. (1965). *The Sexual Behaviour of Young People*. London: Longmans. Also in paperback.

SCHOFIELD, M. (1972). *Sexual Development*. London: The Health Education Council Ltd.

SCHOOLS COUNCIL WORKING PAPER No. 1 (1964). *Science for the Young School Leaver*. Now out of print.

Films

EOTHEN FILMS. 'Man and Woman, Parts I and II,' and 'Childbirth.'

Further Reading

CRELLIN, E., KELLMER PRINGLE, M. L. and WEST, P. (1971). *Born Illegitimate: Social and Educational Implications*. Slough: NFER.
A study of 640 children born out of wedlock in one week in 1958 compared with all other children born in that week, both at the time of their birth and seven years later.

THE FARMINGTON TRUST, 4, Park Town, Oxford, of which John Wilson is the Director. Forthcoming publications include:
For pupils: *First Steps in Morality*.
For empirical researchers: *The Assessment of Morality*. (Conceptual notes on this book, a set of simplified points, are also available.)
For practising teachers: *Practical Methods of Moral Education*.
For young adults and students: *Ideals*.

GOVERNMENT OF THE UNITED STATES OF AMERICA (1971). *Report of the National Commission on Obscenity and Pornography*.
Well researched, but rejected. US embassy library. Bantam Books.

HARRIS, A. (1969). *Questions about Sex*. London: Hutchinson.

HARRIS, A. (1969). *Questions about Living*. London: Hutchinson.

HARRIS, A. (1969). 'Sex education in schools', *New Statesman*, February 28.

THE HEALTH EDUCATION COUNCIL (1971). *Report of the Sex Education Conference at Stamford Hall, University of Leicester*. Copies obtainable from Middlesex House, Ealing Road, Wembley, Middlesex, HA0 1HH.

HYDE, H. (1971). *A Review of Sex Education in Sweden, United Kingdom, Ceylon and Guatemala*.
Dissertation submitted in part fulfilment of the requirement for the M.Ed. (Science Education) Degree of the University of London. Centre for Science Education, Chelsea College of Science and Technology, London SW6.

KIRKENDALL, L. (1968). 'Sex education in research.' *Educ. Res.*, **38**, 5.

NEW YORK BOARD OF EDUCATION (1968). *Family Living, Including Sex Education*. From Board of Education of the City of New York, Publications Sales Office, 110, Livingston Street, Brooklyn, NY11201.
Detailed analysis of concepts and methods from the pre-kindergarten stage to senior high school.

WILSON, J. (1971). A simple introduction to Wilson's work is mentioned in the text, *Moral Thinking*. London: Heinemann Concept Books.
Those who wish a more detailed account should read *Education in Religion and the Emotions*, Chapter 10. London: Heinemann.

WRAGE, E. (1970). *Man and Woman*. London: Collins.
Comprehensive survey including (Freudian) psychosexual aspects from a German Lutheran.